Disability on Equal Terms

Edited by
John Swain and Sally French

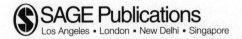
SAGE Publications
Los Angeles • London • New Delhi • Singapore

Contents

Acknowledgements for *Disability on Equal Terms*

Every effort has been made to trace all the copyright holders, but if any have been inadvertently overlooked the publishers will be pleased to make the necessary arrangement at the first opportunity.

Grateful acknowledgement is made to the following sources for permission to reproduce material in this book.

Macfarlane, A. (1994) Watershed, in Keith, L. (ed.) *Mustn't Crumble: writing by disabled women*. London: The Women's Press. Reproduced with kind permission of the author

Cameron, C. (1998) "Sub Rosa" in *Sub Rosa: Clandestine Voices*. Tyneside Disability Arts, Wallsend. Reproduced with kind permission of the author

Sinclair, G. (1999) "Coming Out" in *Transgressions*. Tyneside Disability Rats, Wallsend. Reproduced with kind permission of the author

Higgins, M., and I. Stanton. "Tragic but Brave" http://www.johnnypops. demon.co.uk/poetry/songs/incurables.html

Brisenden, S. (undated) "Scars", from *Poems for Perfect People*. Self-published. http://www.leeds.ac.uk/disability-studies/archiveuk/brisenden/Poems.pdf

Brandon, D. (1990) "Brockhall Hospital" from *Strange Places: experiences in mental handicap hospital*. Salford: University College Salford. Reproduced with permission of the author's estate

Brandon, D. (1981) "The Barrier" from *Voices of experience consumer perspectives of psychiatric treatment*. MIND. Reproduced with permission of the author's estate

Ireland, C. (undated) "Creative Window Truthteller" From the collection *Epochs and Elispe and Epics*, not yet published. Reproduced with kind permission of the author

Introduction

Over the past ten to twenty years there has been a growing literature that has addressed disability from a social model viewpoint, that is analysing the barriers within a disablist society and challenging individual, particularly medical, models that site the problem within the person with an impairment. Such texts can be found throughout the social sciences, some in the arena of sociology, some in disability studies as an academic discipline in its own right, and some directed to specific professional audiences. This book builds on this existing literature but has a particular focus. It sets out to challenge the tragedy model of disability and impairment. It confronts presumptions about disabled people's lifestyles, quality of life, aspirations and needs. In doing so it explores the disablism inherent in western culture, within the disablist language, images and ideologies that are the warp and weft of daily living. It also challenges the professional policy, provision and practice founded in presumptions about disabled people, and looks towards possibilities for change generated by the proud, angry and strong voices of disabled people.

As editors, our starting points came from two directions. The first was the need for a second edition or update of a text edited by Sally French: *On Equal Terms: Working with Disabled People* (1994a). This text has been widely used within disability studies and although the present text is not a second edition, we wanted to retain some of its qualities and aspirations, particularly in addressing the implications for the development of professional services. To signal this we retained the phrase 'on equal terms'. Our second starting point came from the wish to develop the notion of an affirmative model of impairment and disability that we had tentatively explored in previous publications (such as French and Swain, 2004). The imperative to do so comes from many directions. Evidence of the continuing and pervasive dominance of the tragedy view of disability confronts us all again and again. For example, the front-page headline in the *Sunday Times* (5 November 2006) read: 'Doctors: Let Us Kill Disabled Babies'. Whatever the ins and outs of the debate in the report, the headline speaks directly to the crux of the tragedy model: better dead than disabled. The continuing abuse of disabled people was also given some prominence in the front-page *Guardian* headline: 'Catalogue of Abuse in NHS care Homes: Learning disabled were physically and sexually assaulted in units' (17 January 2007). Though these two examples have no direct association, there is a clear association in terms of the treatment of disabled people: killing or abuse.

This new 'on equal terms' book, then, aims to:

- examine the dominant assumptions about disability and impairment and their historical and cultural contexts in western society;
- document the challenges to such presumptions generated by disabled people themselves;
- explore the implication of such challenges for professional policy and practice.

We hope it will be of interest to a wide audience, including disabled people and activists; professionals and policy makers wanting to work on equal terms with disabled people; and degree-level students across a variety of courses. We have purposely brought together a wide range of contributions, including chapters by academics, professionals and researchers, most of whom are themselves disabled. As a consequence, there is a range of styles of writing grounded in personal experience, research and reflections on professional practices.

The social model provides the central consistency in approach throughout this text. Rather than viewing disability as caused by impairment, the social model views disability as resulting from a disabling society in terms of the built environment, the social structures that underpin society and the behaviour and attitudes that disabled people encounter in their interactions with others. The social model thus highlights the social and political nature of disability. In this model disability is viewed as lying outside rather than within the individual, and disabled people collectively constitute a minority group. As with other minority groups, many disabled people have taken the position that disability is a source of both identity and pride, through the celebration of difference. Thus 'disabled people' and 'people with impairments' are the preferred terms in this book as they are used by disabled people themselves for political reasons.

The book is structured in three sections. Each section begins with a chapter by ourselves that sets the scene for the remaining chapters. In **Section I, 'The Tragedy View of Impairment and Disability'**, the chapters explore the tragedy model, the different modes of expression and the consequences for disabled people and their lives. They cover the continuing development of the eugenic ideology, disablist images and language, and the institutional sexual abuse of disabled people. Chapter 1, 'There but for Fortune', sets the scene through an examination of the implications of this model in the lives of disabled people in terms of policy, practice and day-to-day interactions.

The chapters in **Section II, 'From a Different Viewpoint'**, explore the alternative perspectives, that is the non-tragedy view of disability and impairment generated by disabled people themselves. They cover different modes of expression through the collective and individual work of disabled people in a range of art forms and through personal testimony. Chapter 6, 'Affirming Identity', sets the scene by examining the notion of identity and processes of affirmation of disabled identities.

Section III, 'On Equal Terms', takes an innovatory approach to addressing the implications for developing professional policy, provision and practice. The contributors represent a range of health and social care services: occupational therapy, physiotherapy, speech and language therapy, nursing, social work, and also disabled service users/providers. Chapter 11, 'On Equal Terms', sets the scene by highlighting issues of professional power, professional education and the development of services that challenge professional structures and practice. The authors of the remaining chapters were sent a draft of Chapter 11 and were asked to explore the possible implications for their particular professional arena. The result is a collection of pieces that document the mandates and possibilities for changing professional services within professional systems, cultures, power structures and ideologies that have justified, and continue to justify and propagate, the tragedy model of disability and impairment.

Thinking about the project as a whole, for us as editors it is a collective statement. It is a contribution to the literature generated by a social model of disability. It explores the affirmation of disabled identity as expressed by disabled people by all means of communication. It addresses the disability/impairment dichotomy, through affirmation of identities that include impairment and disability. In doing so it documents and analyses the inhuman treatment of people with impairments. It documents too the work of disabled people and their supporters in creating an alternative view of disabled people, their lives and the society in which we all live. It documents the work of professionals committed to realizing and supporting disabled people's affirmative identities.

We would like to thank all the authors who have contributed chapters to this book. They have enabled us, as editors, to develop and deepen our understanding not only of the lives and work of disabled people but also of notions of a society that is fit for all, a society in which disabled people are 'on equal terms' – and we hope you, as readers, will feel you have gained as we have.

Key questions to address

There is now a plethora of literature for health professionals which takes a broadly reflective practice approach, though there are differences between the specific models used. There is also an abundance of courses, both pre-service and in-service, that wholly or partly embrace reflective practice.

The aim of this book is to engage you in critically reflecting on professional policy, provision and practice relating to, and experienced by, disabled people.

This book has been designed as a book to be worked through as well as simply read. In the introductory chapter to each section you will find activities that are aimed at helping you get the most out of the ideas being discussed. A number of processes can be effective and can be drawn on in facilitating critical reflection. We shall outline two: reflective writing and collaboration.

This notion of reflective writing is summarized by Rolfe et al., as follows:

> the reflective writing process is a way of making connections between previously disparate pieces of information, of developing ways of organising or reorganising thoughts, and of exploring issues and structures so as to be able to take a new perspective on them. (2001: 70)

Writing, in this sense, is an active engagement with ideas, a questioning of ideas, a sorting and re-sorting, thinking and rethinking. The activities are prompts, not tests! How you respond is essentially up to you.

The second strategy is collaboration: working with others through the book. This might be a single partner, possibly a colleague or a fellow student, with whom you can engage in the activities, or a series of partners with whom to engage as relevant throughout the book. For us, writing is a collaborative, relational activity, and we are suggesting that reading might be the same for you. The more knowledge and experience is pooled, the richer will be the process of learning. Collaboration requires the establishment of trust in which people can communicate openly and freely.

Section I

The Tragedy View of Impairment and Disability

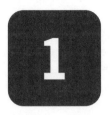

There but for Fortune

Sally French and John Swain

In this chapter the 'tragedy model' of disability, which underpins the topics in this section of the book, will be explored. The main focus of the chapter will be the implications of this model in the lives of disabled people in terms of policy, practice and day-to-day interactions. The tragedy model, as its name implies, depicts impairment and disability as a personal, individual tragedy rather than a social or political issue. As French and Swain state:

In the personal tragedy theory, disability, or rather impairment – which is equated with disability – is thought to strike individuals at random, causing suffering and blighting lives. (2004: 34)

Disability as a tragedy

The tragedy model portrays disability as a biological condition and a limitation (Saxton, 2000), 'as a deficit, a personal burden and a tragedy' (Wilder, 2006: 2), as an enemy (Mason, 2000), as 'abject and abhorrent' (Darke, 2004: 103), and as '"abnormal" and something to be avoided at all costs' (Oliver and Barnes, 1996: 66). Disabled people are perceived as being robbed of any enjoyment in life and as a burden to society (Saxton, 2000). Parens and Asch state:

There are many widely accepted beliefs about what life with disability is like for children and their families … They include assumptions that people with disabilities lead lives of relentless agony and frustration and that most marriages break up under the strain of having a child with a disability. (2000a: 20)

Despite some variation, the tragedy view of disability is widespread across cultures (Coleridge, 1993; Ingstad and Reynolds Whyte, 1995; Stone, 1999a; Barnes and

Mercer, 2005) and throughout history (Stiker, 1997; Longmore and Umanski, 2001; Borsay, 2005) and remains so entrenched in society today that it has become an ideology. Oliver explains that:

> ideologies are so deeply embedded in social consciousness generally that they become 'facts'; they are naturalised. Thus everyone knows that disability is a personal tragedy for individuals so 'affected'; hence ideology becomes common sense. (1993a: 50)

The tragedy model of disability encompasses many perceptions of disabled people, which are nearly always negative. These include notions of inferiority, inadequacy, pity, sadness, evil and disgust. In the Bible, for example, impairment is linked with uncleanliness, sin and possession by devils (Stiker, 1997). Many of the miracles of Jesus (and the antics of recent religious crusaders) concern the curing of impairment, with the implication that disability is both undesirable and tragic. Humphries and Gordon (1992) contend that in the first half of the twentieth century disability was still viewed by many people in Britain as a curse or a punishment. David Swift, who was born in 1936, recalls:

> My grandma used to say that I'd be cursed and I was being punished by God for what I'd done in a past life. That was why I was disabled she said, and when I'd served out this punishment everything would be all right. (1992: 11)

Many disabled children grow up with parents who believe that impairment is a tragedy. This can result in a lowering of self-esteem and in the denial of an important part of their identity. Katrina, a visually impaired woman interviewed by French et al., recalled:

> My mother never accepted me, ever. She couldn't cope with the fact that she had a disabled child. She denied it and expected me to be like everyone else … even when she had reached old age she hadn't accepted it. (2006: 321)

Abelow Hedley recalls her own similar reaction on the birth of her daughter who has achondroplasia (restricted growth):

> When our LilyClaire was born ten years ago, everything was confusion: how to react, how to proceed, what to do. As the frantic first days unfolded it seemed that all we could focus on was how to repair the flaws, and we would listen to anyone from a faith healer to a surgeon if we thought that there was a 'fix' for her in it. I remember thinking: we can put men in space, surely we can fix this. (2006: 43)

Health professionals also have a strong tendency to regard impairment as tragic and undesirable and their power within society has perpetuated this view (French and Swain, 2001). As Morris, a woman born with a Y chromosome and mixed reproductive organs states, 'my diagnosis was considered a tragic mistake of nature by both my physicians and my parents' (2006: 4).

The tragedy media

The words used to describe disabled people are invariably negative or passive. Many words in common use – for example 'short-sighted', meaning lacking in insight – show how deeply rooted negative perceptions of disability are. The very words 'disabled' (not able) and 'invalid' (not valid) indicate the lowly status disabled people have in society. This denigration of disabled people is very widespread. Stone (1999b), for instance, found similar conceptions of disabled people in her studies of ancient Chinese script.

Descriptions of disabled people frequently have tragic overtones, for example 'sufferers' and 'victims', and disabled people are often spoken of as a homogeneous group, for example 'the disabled' and 'the deaf', as reflected in the titles of many leading charities such as the Royal National Institute for the Blind. Disabled people are repeatedly labelled by their impairments ('he's a paraplegic', 'she's an amputee') as if the 'tragedy' of impairment renders everything else about them irrelevant and gives them, as Goffman (1963) explained, a 'master status'. This language also stereotypes disabled people rather than regarding them as unique individuals (Linton, 1998).

The labels ascribed to disabled people sometimes appear, on the surface, to be very positive. For instance, disabled people may be described as cheerful, clever and courageous: indeed, it is not unusual for disabled people to be regarded as courageous simply for living with an impairment, as television programmes such as *Children of Courage* illustrate. The assumption embedded within these 'positive' labels is that disabled people are a group 'apart' who are largely incapable of achieving everyday tasks or attaining a positive state of mind. As a blind physiotherapist remarked:

> *Many people are surprised that we can actually do the job and be good at it. I think it's because they think we are fairly good if we can put one foot in front of the other! (French, 1990: 3)*

In a similar way, parents of disabled children are often perceived as extraordinary and almost saintly, and are commended for 'making light' of disability. Kent, a blind woman, states 'As I was growing up people called my parents "wonderful". They were praised for raising me "like a normal child"' (2000: 57).

The tragedy model assumes that impairment and disability are about loss (with no possibility of gain) and that disabled people, without exception, want to be other than they are (Swain et al., 2003). Keith, who analysed nineteenth-century literature for girls, concludes:

> *The accident or illness in these books is almost always portrayed as a tragedy which must be overcome. The supposition is that the character has become a member of a club that no one wants to join and the corollary is that they start to feel ugly and useless, full of self-loathing. (2001: 222)*

According to Michalko, the perception of disability as tragic is still very prevalent in society today:

> *We are still feared, we are still applauded for simple accomplishments, we are still not the type of person that anyone wants to be, and we are still not welcome. The image non-disabled people have of disability does not yet include any association with 'the good life'. (2002: 12)*

Until recent times disability was defined almost entirely by government, charities, the media and the health professions, all of whom have subscribed to a tragedy model (French and Swain, 2004). This has had serious implications for disabled people in terms of policy and practice. Mason, recalling her times in hospital as a child, states:

> *My memory is basically of a whole series of experiences of being very coldly and formally mauled around. It's very alienating. It's as if you're a medical specimen ... I was never told I was nice to look at or nice to touch, there was never any feeling of being nice, just of being odd, peculiar. It's horrible. It's taken me years and years to get over it. (Sutherland, 1981: 123)*

A central tenet of the tragedy model is that disabled people should strive to be 'normal' and 'independent', whatever the cost to themselves, in order to reduce the 'tragedy' that has befallen both them and their families (French, 1994b). Deaf children, for example, were prevented from using sign language and were punished for using it (Humphries and Gordon, 1992; Dimmock, 1993; Corker, 1996). Lapper, who was born with no arms and short legs, recalls the obsession with 'normality' at the residential home and school she attended:

> *The staff were very keen that we all became proficient in the use of our artificial limbs. The add-on limbs were considered a fundamental aspect of our being able to function properly and fulfil the ultimate aim of the home ... they had great faith in those artificial limbs and thought that if we would only practice and use them regularly we would soon be picking up even the most delicate items without breaking or damaging them. But we all instinctively knew those sorry bits of metal were never going to fulfil their hoped-for potential. (2005: 35)*

Similarly, a disabled woman, talking of her experiences as a patient, states:

> What concerns me most of all is this focus on trying to make me 'normal'. I get that
> from all the therapists. I get a lot of referrals of 'this may help' and 'that may help'.
> They had a massive case conference before the adaptations - it was a case of 'how
> normal can we make her first? Are the adaptations necessary?' (French, 2004: 203)

If disabled people resist these pressures to be 'normal' they often meet with anger and resistance. Sutherland states:

> I've known a few people who, as adults, have refused to walk even though they
> could because it's just not worth the effort. And people have got angry with them,
> often. They've been labelled lazy and all sorts of things. They're definitely
> considered odd if they choose to be in a wheelchair, in the same way that you're
> considered odd if you don't struggle to do something that you can actually do
> even though it takes you six hours. (1981: 69)

The tragedy model in operation

It can be seen that the tragedy model has underpinned a great deal of oppressive policy and practice towards disabled people, some of which will be explored in the following chapters. With the tragedy model in place, there has been no motivation to adjust the environment to take the needs of disabled people into account. The response instead has been to separate disabled people from society and incarcerate them in institutions such as hospitals and residential schools (Ryan and Thomas, 1987; Baker, 1990; Potts and Fido, 1991; Humphries and Gordon, 1992; French et al., 2006). In line with a tragedy model of disability, the rhetoric for the existence of such institutions has often been in terms of 'protection', 'cure' and 'care', ostensibly for the person's 'own good'. Various scandals (Pring, 2003) and disabled people's own accounts tell a different story. Margaret, a visually impaired woman, for instance, relates the practices at her residential school:

> There was another poor girl called Lena. Lena was bent down to the left, she had
> a hearing aid, she was partially sighted, she had heart and lung problems and
> problems with her legs and back. She was very placid and inoffensive but the
> staff really had it in for her. They were absolutely abominable. On walks they
> would taunt her, shouting, 'get a move on!' and call her all sorts of names and
> try to get us to join in. One day she sat down in the middle of the road and
> refused to get up. They poked and pushed her forward and clouted her. She
> hadn't long left the school when she died at 17. I completely believe that they
> killed her. If they hadn't bullied her like that she might not have died. They wore
> her out. They killed her. (French et al., 2006: 328–329)

Similarly, Macfarlane, in her poem 'Watershed', describes the murder of a disabled child in the institution where they were both resident:

> We were quiet hiding our fear
> Knowing in our nine-year-old hearts
> That we were about to witness something
> Frightening and evil.
> One cried quietly,
> And we clutched inadequate towels around our thin bodies
> As Mary, pretty and small, passive and unmoving
> Became the focus of all our attention.
>
> They lifted her effortlessly
> Into the deep porcelain tub
> And then, without warning
> Pushed her pale passive body under the water
> And held her there.
> We felt the fear through our ill-clad bodies.
>
> There was no shriek, no cry, no dramatic action.
> A loud clock ticked on
> A reminder that we had seen this before,
> Had shivered, cried restlessly
> And watched Mary come up again.
> Now we were two weeks more knowing
> And understood that we must not move
> Must not show what we felt.
>
> Mary was dead.
> Her body naked in the porcelain bathtub,
> Tiny, frail, utterly lifeless.
> Her long wavy hair over her face
> Not pretty any more.
> She was so fragile.
> She needed to be hugged, needed to be cared for

But her bathers had no compassion,

They stood motionless over her,

Eyes staring transfixed

Not seeing a human child, not seeing her.

Slowly their attention turned outward to us,

Unacknowledged, unwanted onlookers.

One by one we were wheeled back to our beds

Alone with our fearful thoughts.

No one spoke of Mary again.

It was as if she had never been,

And yet she was our friend,

Part of our lives.

Nearly fifty years later this scene comes and visits me.

Then, we knew we must stay silent.

Now I speak it for all the Marys

In institutions, in hospitals, in segregated schools

And for my nine-year-old self, who had no choice

But to sit and watch. (1994: 161–162)

Because these messages of tragedy, and the behaviour which they induce, pervade society, of which disabled people are a part, it is difficult for them to avoid internalizing the messages and becoming oppressed. As Morris states:

> *Most of the people we have dealings with, including our most intimate relationships, are not like us. It is therefore very difficult for us to recognise and challenge the values and judgements that are applied to us and our lives. Our ideas about disability and about ourselves are generally formed by those who are not disabled. (1991: 37)*

Aspinall articulates the way in which the tragedy view of disability was conveyed to her as a child:

> *the realisation that I had been told lies by those from whom I had a right to expect the truth – my parents – left me sad and angry in equal measure. This breach of trust communicated to me that there was something shameful and unacceptable*

about my body even from those from whom I expected unconditional acceptance.
(2006: 7)

Mason explains:

Enjoyment is the last thing on the agenda when talking about parenting and
disability, but without this the child feels that they are the cause of stress and
anxiety for the people who love them, which of course is another erosion of the
child's self-esteem. Disabled children often learn to be bright and cheerful and
flippant about their own needs as a way of attempting to cheer up their parents.
(2000: 36)

Disabled people frequently find that the non-disabled people around them minimize
or deny their impairments and the disabling barriers they face. This is particularly
damaging for children, as they do not feel accepted by their parents or others whose
role it is to care for them (French, 2004).

Disabled people wishing to become parents have consistently met negative views
of their abilities and the harmful effect that their impairment may have on their children. As Olsen and Clarke state:

Pathology is the perspective typically adopted by researchers looking at
parenting and disability from within clinical disciplines. That is, the incapacity of
disabled parents, and the search for negative outcomes for children of disabled
parents. Studies in the area indicate the degree to which clinical research on
parenting and disability has adopted negative and pathologising frames of
reference. (2003: 7)

Vondra and Belsky provide an example of this attitude to disabled parents:

It is unlikely that an individual who is caught up with his or her own psychological
concerns will have the ability to decenter and take the perspective of the dependent
infant. Without the psychological resources to understand and consequently tolerate
the daily demands and frustrations of an infant or young child (let alone a teenager)
a parent will be hard pressed to demonstrate the patience, sensitivity and
responsiveness that effective parenting requires. (1993: 5)

A user of the mental health services speaks of her experience of this kind of attitude
from a consultant psychiatrist:

I was asking advice on taking medication during pregnancy ... his response to
that was that we shouldn't have children, we'd be passing on defective genes,

and he also said that if I became ill the child would be taken away 'no doubt about it'. (Disability and Difference, 2002)

The tragedy model nearly always underpins research concerning disabled people. This has huge implications for disabled people, as research knowledge frequently forms the basis for both policy and practice. Disability research has typically been medical and psychological in orientation (Barnes and Mercer, 1997; Swain and French, 2004). Even when social research on disability has been undertaken the tragedy view has tended to prevail (Swain et al., 2003).

Charities have been, and are, powerful portrayers of impairment and disability and are strongly rooted in the tragedy model. The images and language that are used have built upon, promoted and helped to create stereotypes of disabled people as dependent and tragic. Hevey examined how charities market particular impairments and concluded that, 'Charity advertising sells fear, while commercial advertising sells desire ... charities promote a brand, not to buy, but to buy your distance from' (1992: 35). Drake (1996) contends that charity advertising presents impairment as undesirable and a personal misfortune and disabled people as helpless, dependent and pitiable, and Barnes believes that, 'By emphasising the "tragedy" of disability these advertisements perpetuate the assumption that living with impairment is a life shattering experience' (1994: 38).

The media (for instance television, radio, newspapers and magazines) are also powerful in portraying disability and impairment and are deeply rooted in the tragedy model (Davies and Pointon, 1997). Barnes et al. (1999) contend that television programmes about disabled people focus mainly on medicine, cure and 'special achievements' and that disabled people are depicted as criminal, powerless and pathetic in order to 'contribute to an atmosphere of mystery, deprivation and menace' (1999: 192). Barnes states that:

> *disability in the mass media is extremely negative. Disabling stereotypes which medicalise, patronise, criminalise and dehumanise disabled people abound in books, films, on television and in the press. They form the bedrock on which the attitudes towards, assumptions about and expectations of disabled people are based. (1994: 45)*

Darke considers that 'the representation of disability in the media in the last ten years is pretty much the same as it has always been: clichéd, stereotyped and archetypal' (2004: 100).

Throughout history and across cultures disabled people have experienced persecution, abuse and discrimination (Oliver and Barnes, 1996; Stiker 1997). The Romans, for example, practised infanticide on disabled infants and in medieval Europe disability was linked with evil and witchcraft, which frequently led to the murder of those convicted (Barnes, 1994). A stark example of the persecution of disabled people in recent European history is the Nazi regime of the 1930s and 1940s that was fuelled by eugenic ideas of 'improving the human race' (Snyder and Mitchell, 2006b). Such ideas were prevalent throughout Europe at this time and were supported by politicians of all persuasions as well as by leading doctors and scientists (Kerr and Shakespeare, 2002; Evans, 2004). Mason states:

> The overall image that was created of disabled people was of being a burden that society could not afford. This reached its peak in Germany in the late 1930s when Hitler's Third Reich issued leaflets comparing the costs of caring for a disabled child with a 'normal' child, proclaiming them to be 'useless eaters'. (2000: 29)

Approximately 375,000 disabled people were sterilized by the Nazi regime between 1933 and 1939, including those with learning difficulties, epilepsy, mental health problems and hereditary deafness and blindness (Kerr and Shakespeare, 2002). Sterilization Acts were passed in many other countries at this time including Finland, Iceland, Sweden, Norway, Denmark, Switzerland and some states of the USA (Evans, 2004). Many of these countries continued to sterilize disabled people until the 1970s and, in the case of Japan, until 1996 (Russell, 1998).

Evans (2004) estimates that approximately three-quarters of a million disabled people were murdered by the Nazi regime, including those with harelips, stutters and minor deformities. So many deaf people were sterilized or murdered that deaf culture in Germany was almost obliterated (Dimmock, 1993; Evans, 2004). Disabled people were also subjected to brutal experimentation before they were killed (Evans, 2004). It is only in recent times, however, that the plight of disabled people under the Nazis has been acknowledged (Morris, 1991). Disabled people were treated unfairly by the courts which meant that very few perpetrators were brought to justice (Russell, 1998; Evans, 2004) and no compensation or recompense has ever been given to those who were sterilized or to the families of those who were murdered (Kerr and Shakespeare, 2002). Kerr and Shakespeare state that:

> A key point to remember about Nazi euthanasia is the central involvement of scientists and doctors. It is impossible to write off what happened as the aberrant behaviour of a group of thugs, fanatics and ideologues. It was doctors, not SS men, who killed in the euthanasia centres or on the children's wards. Prejudice against disabled people, and racial minorities, was enshrined in the scientific orthodoxy of the early twentieth century, and most of those involved in killing and sterilising disabled people felt that they were performing a service both to society and even the individuals themselves. (2002: 44–45)

It can be argued that these negative attitudes and behaviours towards disabled people, underpinned by the tragedy model, still operate in society today in practices such as genetic testing, genetic counselling, abortion of impaired foetuses, genetic engineering and the euthanasia of disabled people.

The Royal College of Obstetricians and Gynaecologists has recently called upon the working party of the Nuffield Council of Bioethics to use active euthanasia on seriously impaired babies, such as those with spina bifida, and has also called for a discussion on the costs of bringing up a severely disabled child (Choppin, 2006). Technology is already in place to screen out impaired foetuses. In a recent newspaper article (Smith, 2006) the mother of twins who undertook this technology to avoid having children with cystic fibrosis states, 'they are designer babies but they are designed for the good of mankind'. Such ideas are being challenged by various groups of disabled people, including the UK group Not Dead Yet, who are opposed to euthanasia and eugenics.

Mason believes that, 'Human genetic engineering is a continuation of the eugenicist belief in social control through manipulation of the gene pool' (2000: 24) and that 'covert eugenic policies still dominate medical practices' (2000: 32). Asch agrees:

> the vast majority of theorists and health professionals still argue that antenatal testing, followed by pregnancy termination if an impairment is detected, promotes family well-being and the public health. To them it is simply one more legitimate method of averting disability in the world. (2001: 306)

Evans sees a direct link between these policies and the Nazi regime:

> The notion of 'imperfect' human beings and the unproductivity and unworthiness of people with disabilities which played such an integral role in Nazi programs, also lies at the root of current policy issues. They form the basis of ongoing debates involving such highly charged topics as gene testing, assisted suicide and the rationing of health care. They creep quietly into policy debates and judicial decisions such as access to insurance and reasonable accommodation in the work place. The discourse on each of these topics is fraught with assumptions about the inherent worth and potential contribution of a person with a disability. (2004: 10–11)

In British law abortion is prohibited after 24 weeks of pregnancy except when the foetus is 'seriously handicapped', when no upper limit is stipulated (Kerr and Shakespeare, 2002).

Conclusion

There are a number of possible explanations of the tragedy model of disability being ingrained within society. According to Oliver and Sapey (1999), non-disabled people have imagined what it must be like to be disabled, have assumed it would be a tragedy, and have decided that it would require a difficult psychological adjustment. Thus non-disabled people have projected their ideas about disability on to disabled people and these, in turn, have been translated into policy and practice. Marks explains that:

> The concept of projection offers one key tool to understanding the psychic mechanisms of prejudice against disabled people ... fears about monstrosity and stupidity can be projected onto disabled people, who are then experienced as threatening or pitiful and who are avoided because they serve as an uncomfortable reminder to non-disabled people of disavowed aspects of themselves. (1999: 23)

This quotation highlights another explanation of the tragedy model: that it reflects a deep irrational fear by non-disabled people of their own mortality (Fawcett, 2000). Hunt, for instance, argues that:

> For the able-bodied, normal world we are representatives of many of the things they most fear – tragedy, loss, dark and the unknown ... contact with us throws up in people's faces the fact of sickness and death in the world ... A deformed and paralysed body attacks everybody's sense of well-being and invincibility. (1966: 155–156)

The fear and discomfort that disabled people induce in others and the ways in which disabled people manage this situation were analysed by Goffman (1963) in his influential book *Stigma*. This has, however, been criticized by disabled people as it assumes that these fears, and the subsequent stigmatization of disabled people, are 'normal' facets of human psychology and behaviour rather than being produced by wide and deeply ingrained social structures (Finkelstein, 1980). A recent example of the fear engendered by illness and impairment, and the hatred, abuse and moral outrage that frequently follow, arose with the occurrence of AIDS (Auto-Immune Deficiency Syndrome) that first appeared in the early 1980s ('Living with Aids: Britain's battle', 2006). Fear can also be a manifestation of ignorance about impairment and disability, which can give rise to feelings of inadequacy about how to communicate with a disabled person or what, if any, assistance to offer (Miller and Sammons, 1999).

A further explanation of the tragedy model concerns the need for human beings to affirm their own identity by comparing themselves with others. Thus the tragedy view of disability serves to confirm that the values of non-disabled people are worthy, good and important. If the disabled person appears to be happy and content this can present an uncomfortable challenge to the values on which the non-disabled person's life is based (Hunt, 1966).

Disabled people throughout history and across cultures have been silenced by powerful organizations and institutions (such as charities, the church, the medical profession and the media) which have defined them and created and maintained their oppressed position within society. Such a long, repressive history, stretching back centuries, is difficult to dislodge, but in recent years, with the growth of the Disabled People's Movement internationally, disabled people are speaking out, writing their own history, analysing their lives, demanding equal opportunities and anti-discrimination legislation and defining themselves in very different ways from those depicted in this chapter. Twenty years ago it would have been very difficult to study disability, as disabled people define it, but now there is an abundance of books and articles on which to draw and Disability Studies, as an academic discipline, has been born. This knowledge, which is constantly developing, is now available to all those who wish to understand the meaning of disability in our own society and across the world.

Some Key Questions to Address in Section 1

Activity

As you read the chapters in this section, collect examples of what you consider to be expressions of a tragedy model of disability and impairment in the media. They may be from newspapers, television programmes (news, documentaries, soaps, comedies, etc.) films, posters (including charity and advertising posters) and so on. With each example reflect on the messages being portrayed about disabled people and their lives, and possible implications for how others think of disabled people and how disabled people think of themselves. We mentioned collaborative learning in the introductory chapter. This activity forms an excellent basis for a group discussion with colleagues or fellow students.

Questions

The chapters in this section explore the dominance of the tragedy model of disability and impairment. As you read spend some time thinking, and if possible discussing, your reactions to this. You might find it helpful to consider the following.

1   The tragedy model is a way of understanding, thinking about and responding to disability and impairment. List assumptions or presumptions that characterize this model.
2   Why is this the dominant model in western societies?

(Continued)

(Continued)

3   The tragedy model reverberates through the lives and experiences of disabled people in numerous ways. List some of the ways it has impinged on and shaped western societies' responses to impairment.

4   A person we interviewed, who was becoming progressively visually impaired in later life, told us that, when she was diagnosed, her doctor had said, 'what do you expect at your age?' This phrase, for us, succinctly conveyed a tragedy viewpoint that incorporated ageism with disablism. It is a recurrent theme in the experiences of older people becoming impaired. It raises questions about the tragedy model in relation to other social divisions, particularly age, ethnicity, gender, type of impairment and sexuality. For instance, the supposed tragedy of becoming impaired can be cast in differing lights for men and women. As you read this section think about the relevance of these other factors in understanding and analysing the expressions of a tragedy model to which disabled people are subjected.

5   Critically reflect on your personal understanding of disability and impairment. It can be argued that we all embrace a tragedy model viewpoint. Indeed, this is part of the dominance of this way of thinking. This can be thought of in at least two ways in relation to non-disabled people. The first is the social context and the ubiquity of expressions of tragedy in images and language – to the extent it becomes 'common sense'. The second is more personal. For a person leading a sighted lifestyle, for instance, the notion of becoming visually impaired can be tragic. At the most extreme it is a fear of our own mortality. As expressed in the title of this chapter: there but for fortune. For some disabled people too, the devaluation may be internalized. Furthermore, many people with impairments do not identify as being disabled and this can, in part, be explained as a denial of the 'disabled' label that carries such negative connotations. Another expression of this is sometimes referred to as a supposed 'hierarchy of disability'. Simply put, this is the notion that some disabled people are 'better off' than others, on the grounds of severity and, sometimes, type of impairment.

The chapters in this section thus provide food for thought in critically reflecting on our own perceptions and presumptions about disabled people and their lives.

2 Disability, Genetics and Eugenics

Tom Shakespeare

In this chapter, I will both review the history of eugenics and look at the long shadow that this story casts over contemporary debates about disability and genetics. Clearly, the eugenic past is relevant to the complex and difficult issues surrounding antenatal diagnosis. Negative thinking about disabled people and reproduction can also be found in other areas of society, and can often be traced back to the eugenic discourses prevalent in previous generations (Snyder and Mitchell, 2006a). Eugenic ideas about the burden of disability, about the dangers of increasing numbers of disabled people, and about the cost to society of supporting disabled people can still be found in popular, policy and biomedical literature. However, most western democratic states make at least a formal commitment to the principles of human rights. The extent to which these principles are fully implemented is variable. Whereas in the early part of the twentieth century, eugenic sterilization was widespread, and indeed continued into the 1960s in some Nordic countries, the practice appears to be uncommon in most contemporary societies, with some exceptions (Dowse and Frohmader, 2001). The obstetrics and genetics professions are based on the principle of informed consent. It is also rare to find individuals being explicitly coerced into testing or selective termination. But there is implicit pressure to avoid the birth of disabled children, as well as wider cultural assumptions that disability is a fate worse than death (Ward, 2001). In some countries, the principle of informed consent is widely ignored (Wertz, 1999).

What is eugenics?

Eugenics cannot be boxed off as a relic of the past. Nor can it be equated in any simple sense with the genetic medicine of the present. But is it possible to come up with a more useful definition? The word itself was coined in 1883 by Francis Galton to mean 'well born'. Galton defined it as 'the science of improvement of the human germ plasm through better breeding'. It could therefore be defined broadly as 'genetic improvement'. This, however, might include a wide range of maternity and paediatric services, possibly the whole of genetic medicine. This stretches the definition of eugenics too far and waters down concerns. Therefore it seems necessary to limit the word to attempts to intervene in the area of inheritance.

The philosopher Jonathan Glover highlights two key definitional parameters on which there seems to be consensus. First,

> If we want to keep the word for the really controversial cases, we can stipulate that a policy is eugenic only if it has the aim of influencing the composition of the population. (Glover, 1999: 116)

Second, Glover expresses a common view in another of his publications, when he specifies further that it is not 'genetic improvement' that is the problem, but the means by which this is achieved:

> Few people object to the uses of eugenic policies to eliminate disorders, unless those policies have additional features which are objectionable. Most of us are resistant to the use of compulsion, and those who oppose abortion will object to screening programmes. But apart from those other moral objections, we do not object to the use of eugenic policies against disease. (1984: 31)

This is the perspective taken by Kevles (1985), when he argues that the contemporary revolution in genetics is not likely to be used for eugenics purposes because of our emphasis on reproductive freedom and civil rights for disabled people, in contrast to the state-sponsored coercion of the past. If we wish to retain a pejorative notion of eugenics, this suggests we could reach a core definition of eugenics as meaning the combination of a population policy to improve the genetic health of the next generation, involving some measure of compulsion. The inhuman dimensions of such an approach lie in the suggestion that individual desires must be sacrificed to a larger public good.

However, problems remain with this approach. First, the historical practice of eugenics included voluntary measures to improve 'racial hygiene' as well as coercion: they also included 'positive eugenics', extra breeding by the 'genetically healthy', as well as 'negative eugenics', less breeding by the 'genetically unfit'. Paul cites the British

Eugenics Education Society, which adopted the tactics of 'education, persuasion and inducement' rather than law or coercion, as in the US model of eugenics (1992: 669). Second, this approach focuses on whether a policy is designed to implement change at a population level: it assumes an agent with a goal. Most modern genetic services are not designed with this explicit intention: instead, they are designed to offer couples choice in reproduction. Yet the outcomes of such an ostensibly non-eugenic approach may be a change in the composition of the population. This is what Duster (1990) has called 'back door eugenics'. The philosopher Kitcher (1996) intends to give a more positive spin to the current western approach of voluntary screening programmes plus reproductive choice by referring to it as 'consumer eugenics'. Caplan et al. (1999) go further, advocating a eugenics that involves enabling individuals voluntarily to enhance the capabilities of their offspring, not just to restore function or correct impairment but actually to improve on their ordinary human capacities. Arguably, these values have much in common with the eugenics of the past, which is why Hampton (2005) has labelled this approach 'family eugenics'.

The era of eugenics

Francis Galton, the founder of eugenics, was a cousin of Charles Darwin, and the ideas of Darwin were a major stimulus to eugenic thinking when it developed in the late nineteenth century, although eugenic ideas actually date back to Plato and the Spartans. Those Victorians and Edwardians who accepted that humans had evolved through natural selection looked at their own society with increasing concern. Many thousands of years of adaptive pressures seemed to be threatened by contemporary developments such as housing and sanitation improvements, welfare reform, and democracy. Whereas in the past, the 'inferior' or weaker human specimens would have died or failed to reproduce, in a more supportive and inclusive society there was nothing to stop them reproducing, according to this viewpoint. This fear of degeneration, like a biological version of entropy, suggested that lower social classes, or inferior races, would come to predominate over 'superior' beings, who were likely to reproduce at a slower rate. Moreover, it was claimed that deleterious mutations were more common than advantageous mutations, so that the population would inevitably decline.

The science underpinning these fears and claims was often highly inaccurate and based on prejudice, not evidence. For example Charles Davenport was Director of the Genetics Laboratory at Cold Spring Harbor, New York and responsible for setting up the Eugenic Record Office in 1910. He claimed that many social differences or traits were hereditary, even the tendency for naval careers to run in families. Like many of his contemporaries, he regarded social behaviour such as alcoholism or promiscuity as inherited biological defects. Another advocate of this unfounded biological determinism was his successor, Harry Laughlin, Director of the Eugenic Record Office, who testified in the United States Congress in 1923 that people from southern Europe were genetically prone to criminality. In the 1930s, Laughlin went on record praising the Nazi sterilization law, and was subsequently awarded an honorary degree from Heidelberg University for his work to promote racial hygiene (Kevles, 1985).

Eugenic ideas challenged the mid-nineteenth-century reformism which had sought to educate and improve the lives of people with learning difficulties. Whereas previously, feeble-mindedness had been seen as part of a continuum of ability, moral entrepreneurs such as Mary Dendy (Jackson, 1996) were now claiming that feeble-minded people were part of a degenerate subset of society, who should be permanently segregated. The idiot was now seen less as 'a challenge for scientific and philanthropic pedagogy than as a burden on the nation' (Rose, 1985: 99). Dendy argued that feeble-mindedness was incurable, and qualitatively different from normality. Segregation would reduce crime, prevent transmission to the next generation, and protect both the individuals concerned and wider society.

The eugenic ideas of Dendy and others were influential on the drawing up of the 1913 Mental Deficiency Act (Jackson, 1996). British campaigners, however, failed to achieve sterilization laws, due partly to the work of libertarian MPs such as Josiah Wedgwood, who called the 1913 Act 'a monstrous interference with individual liberty'. The goals of the eugenic movement, which included voluntary sterilisation of feeble-minded people, and birth control for unemployed workers, had more impact in the United States. Indiana was the first state to pass a sterilization law, in 1907, and fifteen other states followed suit (Kevles, 1985).

While eugenic policies may have had less direct political impact, eugenic thinking was widespread in British society. The novelist Virginia Woolf wrote in her diary for Saturday, 9 January 1915:

> On the towpath we met & had to pass a long line of imbeciles. The first was a very tall young man, just queer enough to look twice at, but no more; the second shuffled and looked aside; & then one realised that every one in that long line was a miserable ineffective shuffling creature, with no forehead, or no chin, & an imbecile grin, or a wild suspicious stare. It was perfectly horrible. They should certainly be killed. (Childs, 2001: 23)

While this may be an extreme example, such attitudes were commonplace at the time. Winston Churchill, MP, had said a few years previously that 'the unnatural and increasingly rapid growth of the feeble-minded and insane classes, coupled as it is with a steady restriction among all the thrifty, energetic and superior stocks, constitutes a national and race danger which it is impossible to exaggerate' and had gone on to propose sterilization to cut off 'the streams of madness' (Thompson, 1998: 33).

Nor were these views restricted to conservative or elitist sections of society. Socialists such as George Bernard Shaw and H.G. Wells were supporters of eugenics. Fabian reformers such as the Webbs wrote pamphlets warning about racial degeneration. The social reformer, sex educator and pro-feminist Havelock Ellis (1927) cited Francis Galton, the father of eugenics. While abjuring compulsory measures such as marriage health licences and sterilization, Ellis claimed that feeble-mindedness was a major problem that arose largely from heredity, not environment. Moreover, feeble-minded people were more likely to reproduce, due to their lack of forethought and restraint. He suggested that:

> It is not only in themselves that the feeble-minded are a burden on the present generation and a menace to future generations. In large measure they form the reservoir from which the predatory classes are recruited. (1927: 37)

By this he meant problems such as prostitution, criminality, vagrancy and alcoholism, concluding that 'Feeble-mindedness is an absolute dead-weight on the race. It is an evil that is unmitigated' (1927: 43).

Prejudice about disabled people found expression and focus in the eugenics movements that flourished in Britain, America, Scandinavia and many other countries at this time. It is not clear whether eugenics was responsible for prejudice against disabled people, or merely gave a pseudo-scientific cover for existing discriminatory views. Clearly, negative views about disability pre-date the late nineteenth and early twentieth centuries. Ideas about racial hygiene and fear about the threat of biological degeneration gave a new impetus for attempts to segregate and control people with learning difficulties, mental illness and threatening behaviours.

From eugenics to genetics

By the 1930s, mainstream eugenics was in decline, to be replaced by what Kevles (1985) labels 'reform eugenics', which in its turn gave way to clinical genetics. After 1945, a realization of the crimes of Nazi racial science led to formal rejection of the aims and terminology of eugenics. For example, Lionel Penrose changed the name of the *Annals of Eugenics* to the *Annals of Human Genetics* in 1954. However, many of the personnel remained the same, and some of the old ideas also persisted.

This period was marked by a repudiation of the old eugenic ideas about selective breeding and a new emphasis on research and statistical analysis by scientists such as Lionel Penrose and R.A. Fisher. H.J. Muller argued that it was impossible to eliminate mental deficiency by negative eugenics, because there might be many unaffected carriers of deleterious genes. Data from intelligence testing showed that average IQ was actually improving, rather than degenerating as the previous generation had feared. The emphasis on racial hygiene was replaced by investigations of health and disease. This research led to better understanding of blood groups, forms of learning difficulties including Down's syndrome and phenylketonuria, and other genetic and developmental conditions.

After the discovery of the structure of DNA in 1953 by Francis Crick and James Watson, genetic science had an understanding of the mechanisms of inheritance which opened up a whole new research agenda. Slowly, clinicians began to be able to offer advice to patients worried about inherited diseases. The new professional field of genetic counselling stressed informed consent as the key value that distinguished the new medical approach from the historical eugenic abuses. From 1960, antenatal diagnosis and selective termination began to become available for a gradually increasing number of conditions.

It would be wrong to conclude that the changed emphasis of genetics necessarily led to changed attitudes by scientists or clinicians. For example, Francis Crick clearly held eugenic views, although he was usually circumspect in expressing them (Ridley, 2006). At the 1963 Ciba Foundation meeting on 'Man and His Future' he argued that people had no right to have children, calling for licensing or taxing of reproduction to discourage breeding among the genetically 'less fit'. In October 1968 he gave the Rickman Godlee Lecture at University College, London. According to the surviving notes of his address, Crick again questioned whether individuals should have the freedom to reproduce; asked whether thalidomide babies should be allowed to live; and suggested it was necessary to promote the quality not just the quantity of children. In a 1970 letter, he suggested bribing individuals who were irresponsible or poorly genetically endowed to be sterilized, a curiously unscientific comment that exactly replicates the sentiments of early twentieth-century eugenics.

James Watson has also often made quasi-eugenic statements. One of his children has a serious mental illness, which appears to have given Watson a very negative and unbalanced attitude towards disability in general. For example, he has written that 'seeing the bright side of being handicapped is like praising the virtues of extreme poverty' (2000: 207). Watson is a libertarian and has objected to state measures to impose eugenic solutions, but he is in no doubt as to the duty of individuals in the realm of reproduction:

> I do not see genetic diseases in any way as an expression of the complex will of any supernatural authority, but rather as random tragedies that we should do everything in our power to prevent. There is, of course, nothing pleasant about terminating the existence of a genetically disabled fetus. But doing so is incomparably more compassionate than allowing an infant to come into the world tragically impaired. (2000: 225)

In 1968, Linus Pauling, the leading biologist and scientific rival of Crick and Watson, famously called for compulsory testing of young people for sickle cell anaemia and other deleterious genes and for them to be tattooed if found to be carriers. Each of these leading scientists appears to have believed that his undoubted expertise in biochemistry and molecular biology gave him the necessary insight, even duty, to pronounce on wider social and political matters.

Eugenic thinking today

The development of clinical genetics and reproductive medicine has privatized eugenics: there has been a move away from explicit population-level policies or coercion, with the focus now on the reproductive decisions of families. There is an extensive debate as to whether clinical genetics and reproductive technology are appropriately labelled as eugenic. One difference is that previous eugenic policies focused on which groups and individuals should be permitted or encouraged to reproduce, while current genetics and reproductive technologies are primarily directed towards avoiding the birth of children with genetic disease. In other words, genetic screening is about which babies people can have, not about which people can have babies. However, the latter concerns do still emerge, particularly in reference to the reproductive rights of people with learning difficulties (Dowse and Frohmader, 2001).

Early twentieth-century concerns about racial degeneration seem ludicrous today. It is clear that the negative thinking about disability that underpinned eugenics remains widespread in certain societies, and can occasionally be seen in most societies. To illustrate the first point, surveys by Wertz (1999) showed that outside Anglo-American societies eugenic ideas remained powerful in thinking about reproduction. In China, for example, this thinking fed through into the Maternal Health Law, which encourages women to avoid having impaired children (Dikitter, 1998). To illustrate the second point, in our British research on sexuality we argued that eugenic fears of disabled people reproducing underpinned some of the prejudice and hostility surrounding disabled people's becoming sexual, and some of our respondents had experienced these prejudices in the responses of non-disabled people to their expressions of love and intimacy (Shakespeare et al., 1996). In the post-war generation, these reactions were even stronger (Humphries and Gordon, 1992).

Looking more closely at contemporary biomedicine, there appears to be an ambivalence about the goals of reproductive and genetic medicine, as expressed in professional and policy statements: often these documents denounce eugenics, while simultaneously suggesting objectives which seem perilously close to pre-war approaches (Clarke, 1991). Lenaghan has suggested that

> *A commitment towards a human rights approach may be used to (cosmetically) distance the speaker from nasty 'eugenic' abuses of genetics without altering the ethos of the service on offer. (1998: 48)*

While the majority of medical professionals may support the principle of informed consent, and disown the eugenic abuses of the past, there are always individuals who are prepared to go on record with atavistic opinions, such as Professor Robert Edwards, one of the pioneers of reproductive technology, who famously announced at a European embryology conference in 1999:

> *Soon it will be a sin of parents to have a child that carries the heavy burden of genetic disease. We are entering a world where we have to consider the quality of our children. (Rogers, 1999)*

Social research has shown that many scientists and clinicians in this field hold views which have eugenic overtones (Kerr et al., 1998). Rarer in mainstream science, but nevertheless persistent, are those whose views explicitly evoke comparison to the racism and anti-egalitarianism of earlier generations, such as the authors of *The Bell Curve*, or the contributors to *Mankind Quarterly* (see Buchanan et al., 2000)

While views on the role of the state versus the individual have changed to the point that it seems unfeasible that western democratic states could subordinate reproductive freedom to racial or population goals, there are inescapable pressures on health care spending and consequent incentives to avoid 'costly' births. For example, discussions of prenatal diagnosis are often couched in the wider economic language of screening, in which cost-benefit analysis suggests that it is worthwhile to introduce public health measures if the cost of detection is less than the cost saved by avoiding the disease (Wald et al., 1992). While understanding the impact and relative priority of different interventions are important, these calculations seem inappropriate and implicitly eugenic in the context of reproductive decisions.

Conclusion

It is easy to denounce historical eugenics, and the more overtly eugenic statements or cost-benefit arguments made in contemporary healthcare fields. It may be harder, however, to reach a consensus on the proper attitude and approach to reproduction or to impairment prevention. Medical attempts to avoid or ameliorate impairment can be challenging to many disabled people. Those who have rejected a view of themselves as limited, invalid or suffering may find it difficult to come to terms with research that promises to remove their impairment, or policies which offer prospective parents the option of avoiding having children like them. Those who have redefined disability as a social creation may find medical responses irrelevant or inappropriate. Those who follow the UK social model conception call for society to be changed, not individuals. Many disability rights activists worldwide believe that the disability difference should be welcomed.

It is not clear how far disabled people in general support this disability movement hostility to impairment prevention and associated biomedical research and practice. Many commentators on the social model perspective have argued that there has been a tendency to ignore the body, and the problematic impact of impairment on the lives of disabled people. Many disabled people are affiliated to groups or organizations that promote medical research on their impairments, such as the Genetics Interest Group or the medical research charities. Others are ambivalent about the issue of antenatal diagnosis and termination of pregnancy, challenging the cultural tendency towards identifying and eliminating foetuses with impairment, while not criticizing the decisions of individual prospective parents. Those who support a woman's right to choose have a difficult task in defending the principle of abortion rights in general, but opposing the choice of termination on the grounds of foetal abnormality in particular.

Expressivism is the key argument used by disabled activists and academics seeking to challenge contemporary antenatal diagnosis and subsequent parental choice to terminate pregnancies on the basis of foetal abnormality. The expressivist objection suggests that these policies and practices are objectionable because they express negative views of disabled people. The effect of selective termination is to suggest that disabled people's lives are not worth living, or that disabled people are less worthy than other members of society. As Asch has argued:

> Do not disparage the lives of existing and future disabled people by trying to screen for and prevent the birth of babies with their characteristics. (Parens and Asch, 2000b: 13)

The force of the expressivist objection is in highlighting the negative cultural imagery and language that surround the offer of antenatal diagnosis, and society's wider views of the desirability of avoiding impairment at all costs. The debates and literature about genetics and other preventative health measures often perpetuate very negative images of disabled people and messages about disability. If people are to exercise choices, they must be able to do so in contexts that are respectful and welcoming of disabled people. This means challenging the assumption that disability is inevitably a tragedy, but also ensuring that better services and support are available for disabled people and their families. This enables prospective parents to continue pregnancies knowing that the society their children enter will be committed to inclusion and equality.

Many researchers have demonstrated that prospective parents are denied full information, proper support and a real choice in whether to have testing, and whether to terminate (summarized in Shakespeare, 2005). Without full consent and balanced information – in particular, about the nature and impact of impairment – antenatal screening comes perilously close to eugenic abuse. Specific measures that could make choice more real include better training for medical and nursing staff about disability, and more balanced representations of disabled lives – such as my own team's initiative to produce the Antenatal Screening Web Resource (www.antenataltesting.info).

Whereas the expressivist objection is a useful and timely challenge to the ethos of screening, in my view it does not suggest that antenatal diagnosis or selective termination is necessarily wrong in all cases, or should be prohibited. Here I think we need a debate about the nature of impairment itself, a debate that the disability movement has often tried to avoid. Impairment is very varied, ranging from minor anomalies or difficulties to much more serious conditions which cause pain, suffering and extensive restriction. While genetic advocates like James Watson make the mistake of assuming that all impairment is appalling, disability rights advocates sometimes make the opposite error of thinking impairment is just another difference. James Watson ignores the fact that many people with many different impairments lead good, full lives which are not determined or destroyed by suffering. Some activists ignore the very serious diseases such as Lesch-Nyhan syndrome, Tay-Sachs disease, epidermolysis bullosa and other conditions that truly seem to result in a life that, I believe, no human being should have to lead. It is my contention that impairment is rarely neutral: elsewhere, I have suggested that we should think of disability as a predicament, a word which is less negative than tragedy but still captures the challenge that impairments often make to people's lives (Shakespeare, 2006).

It is my own view that we need a medical approach that respects disabled people and disability equality while seeking to minimize the impact of impairment. In general, individuals usually want to avoid impairment in themselves and in their children, where they can, and this does not necessarily reflect hostility to disabled people. Resorting to emotive rhetoric about eugenics and conspiracies to eliminate disabled people seems to me unhelpful (Shakespeare, 1999). It is necessary to work towards a more complex and nuanced view of impairment and genetics.

At the same time, work to combat disability discrimination should be our main priority. It does not seem to me incompatible to support prevention of both impairment and disabling barriers. There will always be disabled people in the world, because disability is part of the human condition. Congenital impairment comprises 1–2 per cent of all births, whereas most estimates place the number of disabled people in society at between 10 and 20 per cent, depending on definitions. Half of all disabled people are older people. This indicates that no amount of antenatal diagnosis will eliminate disability, and that it is imperative to remove barriers and promote equality in order to mitigate the consequences of impairment and improve the quality of life of disabled people.

Both sides of the argument have a responsibility to encourage/promote more careful discussion of the complex issues around genetics and screening. The ultimate decisions about testing and termination should be left to prospective parents, but we can ensure that the context in which they make their choices is respectful of us as disabled people, and our contribution to society. Eugenics did not cause disability prejudice, but it certainly reinforced, sustained and exaggerated it in the early part of the twentieth century. Understanding that history is necessary for those seeking to develop genetic medicine and improve human health in the twenty-first century.

3 Disabled in Images and Language

Margaret Taylor

Everyone who is born with an impairment or who lived as a non-disabled person before becoming disabled is submerged in disablist images. These can be seen as the product of a society founded on the segregation of disabled people. Fundamental to this is the use of images either for dramatic purposes (such as people with visual impairments used for humour) or for charity purposes that promote fear or pity of disabled people and impairment. Lens-based media have facilitated this objectification of disabled people through the manipulation of their image, justifying this on the grounds of simple expediency: 'the camera never lies'. This power of the photograph, film and television to persuade through apparent authenticity has ensnared disabled people in a tragedy model of impairment that has determined perceptions of impairment for non-disabled and disabled people alike for decades. It is only in recent years that some examples can be found of a growing sensitivity to the representation and inclusion of people with impairments in the mainstream mass media. This chapter recognizes the primacy of the image in promoting the values of contemporary culture; outlines the origins and history of the representation of disabled people; and analyses some new imagery that has appeared since the millennium and that marks a greater awareness that ownership of such images must rest with disabled people themselves, and a commitment to achieving this.

Academic analysis of images of disability in the media only began to appear in the early 1990s. However, there is now a significant literature that addresses the representation of disabled people in literary and visual forms, including TV, film and the media (Morris, 1991; Hevey, 1992; Cumberbatch and Negrine,

(Continued)

(Continued)

1992; Norden, 1994; Shakespeare, 1994; Pointon and Davies, 1997; Barnes et al., 1999; Barnes and Mercer, 2003). Historically, disabled people have always been perceived as providing 'rich' subject matter for spectacle, curiosity and metaphor, but the authority of the image in encoding and endorsing generalized and negative perceptions of impairment escalated throughout the twentieth century as the technologies of photography, cinema and television developed. Hughes refers to this 'ocularcentric culture', describing its 'preference for physical and mental perfection [as] … a source of aesthetic discrimination that invalidates and excludes people with impairment' (2002: 580). Giddens similarly describes disabled people as having been 'lost' behind images over which they have had no control, in a 'society dominated by appearances' (1991: 172).

The photographic shaping of impairment

Photography, from its inception, supplied tangible images that could function as a focus for the voyeuristic gaze and position the disabled person as 'other'. The *carte de visite* produced in the mid-nineteenth century as a souvenir of a visit to a circus or 'freak' show provides as early example of the ways in which disabled people were manipulated through their images (Pultz, 1995; Bogdan, 1996; Ostman, 1996). A variety of devices were employed to intensify the image of impairment and construct and manipulate identity in terms of this single defining feature. This might involve, for example, placing the disabled person against a domestic backdrop to heighten and contrast difference. People of contrasting stature were posed together to maximize their disparity, and it was common practice to aggrandize the social position of the subject by using absurdly inflated titles such as *Captain*, *Princess* or *King* (Bogdan, 1996: 29). Thus in a 1915 postcard representation of a woman of restricted growth, a vase of flowers of similar size is placed beside her with the caption, 'Princess Wee Wee the smallest perfectly formed little woman in the world'. The anecdotal text that directs comments in a familiar or sensationalist 'aside' to the viewer becomes an enduring device in the objectification and exclusion of disabled people, appearing later in tabloid newspapers and television documentaries.

Photography, which it was believed offered empirical, objective knowledge, was notoriously at the centre of scientific initiatives to classify physiognomy and impairment, as well as central to the Nazi promotion of the classical 'Aryan' body. Barnes and Mercer (2003), Edwards (1992), Ewing (1994) and Evans and Hall (1999) describe how the medical model of disability was authenticated through documentation facilitated by new photographic technology. This systematic separation, sorting and classification of impairment is characteristic of the Modernist approach to rationality and order and it was used extensively to collect documentary evidence of people with impairments and people of non-western ethnicity. This collection was made in the belief that 'the type, the abstract essence of human variation could be perceived as an observable reality' (Edwards, 1992: 7). The ensuing images, intended as an objective record of impairment or ethnicity, resonate with the social, political and moral ethos of the age.

Charity advertising

Hevey's (1992) analysis of images of disabled people produced as part of the charity advertising campaigns of the 1980s is seminal. These oppressive images left an enduring legacy whereby negative and limiting perceptions became synonymous with impairment and disability. In the 1980s and 1990s there was a shift in emphasis towards a greater reliance on private charity organizations. As these organizations grew into multibillion-pound businesses, fierce competition to boost products in an intensifying market economy meant that professional advertising agencies were employed to use the same devices that large corporate companies adopt to sell their products. In charity advertising, tragedy, pity and helplessness were promoted on the basis that these were the necessary prerequisites for giving.

The impairment became the 'unique selling proposition' for the charity product, in a construction that represented disabled people as a particular kind of person subject to a process of 'image specialisation' (Evans and Hall, 1999: 279). The disabled person had become a commodity owned by the charity. Charities 'marketed' them in the context of assumed negative public perceptions, counteracting this with text that implied superior specialized understanding and knowledge. For example an image of a young person in a wheelchair reaching for the buttons that operate a lift is accompanied by text that presumes to represent her voice: 'Everyone assumes I won't want to get to the top.' The Spastics Society at the bottom of the poster 'answers' her, and us, with the response: 'Our biggest handicap is other people's attitude' (Hevey, 1992: 11). Hevey describes the production of such images as a closed circuit process employing non-disabled people appealing to a public assumed to be non-disabled and bypassing disabled people completely.

Charity advertising assumed that people with impairments belonged to a homogeneous dependent and powerless group. A number of devices which Evans and Hall refer to as 'the various paradigms of the signifying tool kit – clothing, lighting, camera angle, facial expression etc. – were employed in the construction of disabled people as "outsiders"' (1999: 281). The use in early charity images of stark, grainy, black and white photographs taken with deep shadows set the subject apart in a world drained of the colour used to signify the richness and vibrancy of experience that the rest of society can anticipate. Monotone created the alienated shadowy ambience of someone that Hevey describes as 'neither dead nor alive, neither out of society nor in it' (1992: 34). To achieve greater pathos a child was often depicted in these advertisements and in the case of the Royal National Institute for the Blind an atypical, small, totally blind child reading Braille would be depicted when in reality the majority of visually impaired people are, of course, over 75 and not totally blind. It is also interesting to note the Guide Dog Association's recognition of society's greater susceptibility to the appeal and 'pulling power' of Labrador-type dogs rather than visually impaired people. They have always focused on the dogs rather than the people in their imagery.

These images encouraged the observer to 'look in' benevolently at the disabled person's predicament. Their gaze is not returned, allowing avoidance of disturbing notions of individuality and personality. Shakespeare compares the objectification of disabled people in charity advertising with the objectification of women in pornography in the sense that 'in each case, the gaze is focused on the body, which is passive and available' (1994: 288). He suggests that 'in each case the viewer is manipulated into an emotional response: desire, in the case of pornography, fear and pity in the case of charity advertising'.

Resistance by disabled people to 'charity as an agent of dependency' was expressed by an increasingly vociferous lobby against charity appeals such as Comic Relief, BBC Children in Need, Live Aid and the Thames Telethon (Hevey, 1992: 26). The much-publicized 1990 picket of Telethon drew between 150 and 250 disabled demonstrators protesting against the representation issue from the social view of disablement. Hevey describes how this highlighted the growing conflict between the charity advertising representation of disablement and the growing presence of a political body of disabled people seeking access and rights.

Representation in film and on television

Norden considers film the 'most pervasive and influential of the media arts, functioning as a reflection of the values of the society from which it has arisen, and which society then takes up in an unquestioning way and reaffirms' (1994: 1). Certainly cinematic technologies have raised the quality of image and sound to make film a 'particularly intense experience' for the audience (Abercrombie, 1996: 10). Traditionally, impairment has been used to enrich this narrative, based on the long association of good and bad with particular physical characteristics. It has served as a metaphor for a variety of moral statements in stereotypes so durable and pervasive that, for people with and without impairments alike, they became the authentic model of disability. These characterizations, which Norden summarizes, include bitterness, loneliness, courage and triumph (against extraordinary odds), 'violence prone beasts', comic characters, saintly sages and 'sweet young things whose goodness and innocence are sufficient currency for a one-way ticket out of isolation in the form of a miraculous cure' (1994: 3).

The representation of people with impairments as the villain, or the personification of evil, has been a compelling and enduring motif for filmmakers, reiterating the perception that 'deformity of the body is a sure sign of deformity of the mind' (Norden, 1994: 32). From the 1930s onwards increasingly sophisticated special effects endorsed this association, notably in Charles Laughton's portrayal of *The Hunchback of Notre Dame* (1939), the evil megalomaniacs of the 1960s James Bond films, and the fantastical figure of Darth Vader in the 1980s film, *Star Wars*. Literature, which has provided the narrative for many films, also has a history of manipulating the association of impairment with malevolence, from Shakespeare's Richard III to Disney's Captain Hook.

The film industry has seldom, if ever, represented disabled people as sexual beings, recognizing that romance, sexuality and impairment have always been taboo or controversial issues. Impairment has been used more readily as a metaphor for dependency and vulnerability and as a vehicle for exploring such experiences, particularly from the male perspective (Morris, 1991). Gender stereotyping has meant that disabled men have been significantly more in evidence in films than women. Dependency and vulnerability have traditionally been associated with femininity, regardless of impairment. However, the relationship between physical attractiveness, sexuality and impairment disqualifies disabled women on the basis that their impairment, in conventional terms, renders them sexless, with the exception of women with learning difficulties who are often thought to be promiscuous.

Two films that are ostensibly about disability, *My Left Foot* and *Born on the Fourth of July*, Morris describes as actually being about the horror for men of physical and emotional dependency. She states: 'the films rely on the general association of impotence with disability, and on the association of heterosexuality with a stereotyped masculinity' (1991: 94). Paradoxically, even roles that require the characters to be disabled have invariably been played by non-disabled actors, and disabled people seldom appear in roles where their disability is a secondary characteristic. It would seem that directors have been reluctant to cast disabled people in such roles, perhaps because they lack the necessary training and experience, which traditionally have been either inaccessible or simply not considered appropriate for disabled people. An even greater influence has been the powerful meaning that is given to visible impairment on the screen.

Abercrombie states that 'some 97% of households own at least one television set, with television watching occupying more time than all other leisure pursuits combined'. He suggests this implies that television is 'perhaps the most important source of common experience for the British people' (1996: 2) and would 'seem to be describing the world as it is'. This 'world', according to Cumberbatch and Negrine's (1992) detailed analyses, does not include disabled people who, they found, were under-represented or absent across the range of television genres and who, when they had appeared, were portrayed in particular and limiting ways. Morris commented, at the beginning of the 1990s, 'I could watch television for years, possibly a lifetime, without seeing my experience reflected in its dramas, documentaries, news stories' (1991: 84).

Throughout the late 1990s, the presence of disabled people on television was largely limited to 'specialist' disability programmes in off-peak slots. However, disabled people appeared and continue to appear in mainstream programming as part of charity appeals, human-interest stories on local news programmes and particularly in documentaries that explore medical and social narratives. These documentaries, as like the photographic image at the beginning of the century, allow the audience an opportunity to gaze as detached spectators in the privacy of their own homes. The voice-over continues with the aside that addresses the non-afflicted in ways that assume certain values. This style of programme which features disabled people successfully fitting into a 'normal' life or achieving 'against all odds' began to appear as the generation of thalidomide babies grew up from the 1960s onwards, and has found its apotheosis in BBC 1's reality-style series *Beyond Boundaries* which started in October 2005. In this the audience are invited to 'imagine being abandoned in a remote South American jungle and having to fight [their] way across 220 miles of rough terrain'. They are then further invited to 'imagine the added difficulty of completing that journey if [they] are seriously physically disabled' (Elliott, 2005). This endurance test for disabled people was considered sufficiently appealing and sensationalist to be scheduled in mainstream peak viewing time.

The programme focused specifically on a group of disabled people as they endeavoured to meet the challenges set by their non-disabled executive producer who claimed that the intention was to 'inspire everyone through their courage' (McIver, 2005). The admiration that is prompted by participants' bravery and determination is enlivened by the anticipation of who will be the next to have to give up through sheer physical exhaustion or illness. This exclusion clause, which is central to reality TV shows such as *The X Factor* and *Big Brother*, leaves only those whom disabled people label, in a parody of non-disabled perceptions, as 'super crip' (Pointon and Davies, 1997: 81). The reality TV formula of placing together diverse groups of individuals in difficult situations to provide entertainment from the resulting discord creates, in *Beyond Boundaries*, disabled 'heroes' and 'villains'. The notion of 'heroism' or 'saintliness' being associated with disabled people simply by virtue of their impairment is similarly endorsed in programmes such as BBC's *Children of Courage*. Disabled children are given awards because of their 'bravery in the face of disability' alongside children who for instance have rescued people from burning houses, (*Daily Mail*, 14 December 2005).

Documentaries such as Channel 5's *Extraordinary People* and Channel 4's *Born to be Different* (November 2005) rely on the old formula of combining scientific medical procedures with highly personalized and emotive narratives that merge notions of tragedy with hope, and of spectacle with medical enquiry. Described by the programme makers as 'inspiring and sometimes heartbreaking but always thought provoking' (website, Channel 5 2005) a sympathetic response is encouraged from the viewers who, from the implied superiority of their own condition, can indulge in the 'emotional enjoyment of their generous sympathy' (Pointon and Davies, 1997: 141).

The titles, with their invitation to view 'The Woman with Half a Body', 'Joined at the Head' and 'The Girl whose Muscles turned to Bone' objectify disabled people in ways used to bring in the punters in nineteenth century freak shows (Channel 5, *Extraordinary People*, November 2005). The emphasis in such programmes is on the resources employed to remedy or 'normalize' the situation with little reference made to social arrangements, attitudes and values and the bearing that these have on the disablement of the impaired individual.

The impact these ways of representing disabled people has had on disabled and non-disabled people is difficult to measure. Gauntlett and Hill's research is guarded about the extent to which people's individual identities are affected by watching television. However, they made an exception with the disabled participants in their research where they reported people 'making connections between their personal identities and media representations' (1999: 133). They reported concerns that television should 'reflect [disabled people's] lives in a fair and unsensationalized way' for their own sense of identity as well as other people's perception of disabled people. Self-esteem was similarly undermined by the tenor of programmes that were designed to elicit an emotional response. Where donations were generated as a consequence this was resented and seen as an excuse for inadequate government funding.

Cumberbatch and Negrine (1992) saw the hierarchical organization of television and its economic structures as barriers to any changes in the representation and inclusion of disabled people. By the end of the 1990s, however, Gauntlett and Hill were more optimistic. 'Identity politics has made familiar a list of categories – gender, ethnicity, sexuality, disability and (to a lesser extent) age which are now "up for grabs" in identity terms' (1999: 132). This was certainly borne out by programmes such as *Freak Out* (Channel 4, 2000) and the BBC 2 (2002) season of broadcasts *What's Your Problem?* that Gauntlett and Hill describe as intending to reflect the disability experience by 'challeng[ing] traditional assumptions about the supposed markers of identity, and ally[ing] themselves instead with new social movements or new modes of everyday lifestyle' by offering a 'selection box' of identities and 'ways of living and being in the world' (1999: 132).

In an interview in 2000, Channel 4's disability adviser highlighted this new approach to disability programming, describing how 'everyone [commissioning editors] is now encouraged to "own" disability, rather than having disability programmes coming out of only one department' (Minty, 2004). Alison Walsh states: 'we have moved away from the idea of the non-disabled film-maker peering in at the life of a disabled person some years ago. It is the disabled person's take that we are interested in.' This is certainly true in programmes such as *The Boy Whose Skin Fell Off* (Channel 4, March 2004) and *Every Time You Look at Me* (BBC2, April 2004). In these programmes the subject, or actors involved, collaborated with the filmmaker, in the first instance to create an account of living with impairment, and, in the second, to act as consultants in the scriptwriting. The results were positive in that, in the former, stereotypical responses of pity or helplessness were forestalled despite the graphic representation of an impairment that had profound implications; and, in the latter, the notion of disabled people as asexual was challenged whilst the difficulties inherent in a relationship between two people who have a physical impairment were acknowledged, not least their struggle with internalized stereotypical and oppressive perceptions of disability (Mickery, 2004).

However, whilst stating her intention to try and revolutionize television in terms of how they see and deal with disability, Walsh conceded that this task is compounded by the need to change how television currently operates in terms of the personal recommendations, nepotism and referrals that Cumberbatch and Negrine highlighted in 1992. She admitted that 'commissioning editors under a lot of pressure to make progress on multicultural diversity, tend to make disability the second phase of the great diversity battle'. She also expressed concerns that disability was doomed to be a 'string of brave new experiments' and she was aware that the barrier that seems to prevent directors casting disabled actors in roles not actually written as disabled has yet to be broken.

Darke suggests that the 'mainstreaming of disability' has had negative consequences for the representation of disabled people in the media. He argues that impairment imagery, within the specialist disability television programmes, is more than ever 'linked to a charity or "freak" philosophy [that is] fundamentally voyeuristic and exploitative' (2004: 100). He suggests that a significant depoliticization of disability has taken place, with political significance replaced by political correctness: 'the language has changed but not the politics behind it'. He describes this growing political correctness as a sanitizing process which masks the fact that there is still little understanding of the 'genealogy of oppression through culture' and that a distinction has arisen between what he describes as the 'normalized' and the 'un-normalizable' disabled person; 'the "good" and the "bad" cripple' (2004: 101).

In contrast Hughes sees the emergence of a post-modern change of mood, as a 'counter culture' that is

> first and foremost a celebration of difference, a festival of despised identities, a coming out of all those unruly elements who refused to be purified, suburbanised, made into the image and likeness of a sterile and unimaginative sense of responsibility, and an overbearing sense of order and duty. (2002: 578)

He describes modernity as starting to 'dissolve, or rather show signs of a condition of post modernity within itself': 'The stranger could be cool and disorder could be interesting or pleasurable.'

Fashion and lifestyle

This concept of the 'stranger as cool' has been explored in a radical initiative led by fashion designer Alexander McQueen. In this, disabled people had glamorous clothes designed especially for them that they then modelled for a fashion shoot by Nick Knight. These images, which were featured in the style magazine *Dazed and Confused* (no. 46, September 1998), challenged fashion conventions, notions of ugliness, beauty, fantasy and reality and the traditional associations that accompany representations of disabled people. They were considered sufficiently iconic to appear as a banner in the Turbine Hall of Tate Modern (Spring, 2001) but achieved little in the way of removing the difficulties that disabled people face in maintaining such a presence in the fashion industry. According to Knight, 'the industry responds [to intense economic pressure] by appealing increasingly to the mainstream … anything even slightly out of the ordinary frightens people' (*Guardian Weekend*, 29 August 1998).

'Lifestyle' has taken on particular significance in modern social culture, with leisure and sport seen as an important marker of identity and status in late twentieth-century culture and society (Barnes et al., 1999). High profile celebrity status for some notable disabled athletes like Tanni Grey-Thompson has provided role models and celebrity prestige by inference for disabled young people. A number of initiatives also appeared at the end of the 1990s in an attempt to counter discrimination and represent disabled people more fully. Eagle (2003), then Minister for Disabled People, reported that both government and advertising industry professionals were beginning to 'get to grips' with the concepts behind the Images of Disability Initiative and that in 2003 half of all new government advertising campaigns included disabled people. Early examples of this government-backed campaign featured a series of DfEE posters that parodied stereotypical responses to disability. These, however, have been subsumed by the inclusion of disabled people without reference to their impairment.

From 2000 onwards, a flurry of advertisements appeared that included disabled people (Lloyds Bank, British Telecom and McDonald's, January/February 2000). From 2002 the frequently seen 'link' between BBC programmes that highlights different dancers and dance styles has included three wheelchair dancers. Most notable, however, was the Internet provider Freeserve's advertisement featuring Aimee Mullins (Channel 4, June 2000). Mullins, who had appeared on the front cover of *Dazed and Confused* as part of the McQueen project, challenged conventional notions of prosthetic limbs with her glamorously realistic 'mannequin legs', complete with nail varnish and with an alternative pair of bespoke carbon-fibre, curved prosthetics which enable her to move with speed and grace. The advertisement created an impression of style and power by interspersing shots of a leopard running with Mullins's appearance on the catwalk wearing a dazzling feline mane. As she moves from walking to running, the applause of the audience matches her increasing speed and confidence. This inspired advertisement marked a break through in the long history of oppressive imagery of disabled people, with a representation that recognized the strength and beauty of the whole person, providing a role model that added some much-needed glamour to the representation of disabled people.

The inclusion of disabled people in the advertising campaigns of big corporations acknowledged them as potential consumers and as contenders in the process of buying into an 'exciting' and 'aspirational' lifestyle. This is, as for everyone else, a mixed blessing. Celebrity has been achieved by a small but growing number of people with impairments (Matt Fraser, Aimee Mullins, Shanon Murray, Ade Adepitan) all of whom can, despite their impairments, be seen to meet conventional standards of attractiveness. Barnes et al. point to 'the dangers of the advertising industry moving from selling the beautifully sculptured non-disabled body to selling the beautiful and sculptured disabled body' (1999: 196).

Darke is more emphatic in his condemnation of such notions of 'positive' images and the role that they play in reinforcing the dichotomy he perceives in current representations of disabled people in the media, as the 'good and bad cripple scenario'. This he sees as 'the enhancement of the normalized disabled person over and above the valuation of disabled people *per se*'. He states:

> One has only to think of the pretty Para-Olympian or the pretty disabled ex-model
> or dandified karate-kicking disabled television presenters, who the main charities
> use in their advertising, in order to see their increasing dominance as the (stereo)
> type used in the 'positive' representation of disabled people on television.
> (2004: 103)

His concern focuses on the ambiguity he associates with these disabled celebrities: that they are seemingly politicized whilst, he suggests, 'entirely wrapped up within the mainstream oppressive structures of media and charity alike' (2004: 103).

Gauntlett and Hill suggest that 'the validation of complex identities is currently acting as 'merely a springboard for the imagination', and is still in its infancy (1999: 132). Hughes warns that judgement on the depth of post-modern tolerance must be qualified by the acknowledgement that there are 'still barriers, places and spaces where disabled people cannot go' (2002: 580). This is epitomized by the debate generated in the media (March 2004), concerning whether the fourth plinth in Trafalgar Square is the 'right' place for Marc Quinn's 4.7-metre-high marble sculpture entitled 'Alison Lapper pregnant'. This work was created as part of a series of marble sculptures of disabled people born without limbs or who have lost their legs or arms because of accident or illness. Quinn (2002), who had observed people looking at fragmented sculptures in the British Museum, realized that the reaction of the visitors would be the exact opposite if they confronted real limbless people.

The decision to install Quinn's statue generated a mixed response. The work was viewed positively as having 'extraordinary artistic value and merit' which would, with its focus on questions of idealism, heroism, femininity, prejudice and identity,' enhance London's reputation as a leader in the visual arts (Hilty, 2004; Nairne, 2004). Criticism focused on the appropriateness of the location, i.e. Trafalgar Square, which, it was argued, ought to reflect the great moments in history as represented by its current, more illustrious occupants (Hattersley, *Daily Mail*, 17 March 2004). Quinn believed that, in contrast to the dominant, triumphant, male statuary that celebrates the conquering of the outside world, the statue of Lapper represents a new model of female heroism and the contemporary challenge to conquer personal circumstances and the prejudices of others. The fact of her pregnancy makes this a monument to the future (Quinn, 2002).

Conclusion

It is unclear how these contemporary representations of people with impairments will develop and cohere with the emerging cultural analyses within disability studies and disability arts. Darke (2004) argues that the representation of disabled people currently is much as it has been for the last ten years, namely 'clichéd, stereotyped and archetypal'. However, mainstream producers of imagery in the mass media have at least become more aware of the ways in which disabled people are represented and have become more committed to an inclusive approach.

This chapter has traced the ways in which historically images have endorsed and emphasized the social construction of disability, perpetuating negative and oppressive perceptions that have dominated the representation of disabled people up until the turn of the century. The cultural exclusion of disabled people has been challenged by the disability movement and disability arts, and as a consequence, supported by government initiatives, new and inclusive ways of representing disabled people in the mass media have begun to appear in recent years. As yet these do not represent a substantive response to the inclusion of disabled people across all mainstream cultural contexts, but rather a conscious response to the diversity agenda. Unresolved questions of culture and identity that have arisen from the social model of disability are made more complicated by a complex, rapidly changing and consumer-driven society that presents a challenge to disabled and non-disabled people alike in the expression of human diversity and the recognition that we are all part of a spectrum of difference.

4 Institutional Abuse

Colin Goble

In this chapter I will explore the origins and nature of the 'institutional abuse' of disabled people, with particular reference to people with learning difficulties. I would stress here that when using the term 'abuse' I do not mean sexual or violent physical abuse, perpetrated by rogue carers and/or others, though this has certainly been a feature of the experience of institutional living for many disabled people. Rather, I mean the pervasive violation of the right of disabled people to experience the same quality of life as other 'non-disabled' citizens; a form of discrimination akin to institutional racism or sexism.

Institutional forms of 'care' have historically been one of the main models of service provision for disabled people in the UK and across the developed world. In recent decades we have seen a shift towards 'community care', which, for people with learning difficulties in particular, has meant either continuing to live in their family (usually their parents') home, or state, voluntary or private sector residential services provided in small-scale housing or 'hostel' type accommodation. The move towards this form of provision was seen as important in bringing to an end 'institutionalized' models of care. Research into the reality of community-based services has shown that this hope was naïve, and that institutional models of care, and institutional abuse, have been remarkably persistent (Johnson and Traustadottir, 2005). It is my intention to explore some of the reasons why this is so, with a central argument being that this form of abuse is often an integral part of institutional models of care, regardless of whether the actual setting is a large isolated hospital, or a typical suburban house. At the root of this model of care, and of the abuse to which it frequently gives rise, lies a persistent 'pathologization' of disability that often continues to dominate perceptions of disability held by staff and health and social care staff and professionals, despite rhetorical assertions to the opposite. I will illustrate the impact of this form of abuse by looking at the way it impacts on service response to the health of people with learning difficulties.

I will begin by briefly outlining the history of the institutional care of people with learning difficulties. Similar histories could be outlined relating to the institutional care of people with physical and sensory impairments. I have chosen to look specifically at people with learning difficulties, partly because this is the history most familiar to me, but also because, arguably, no other group has been quite so thoroughly and repeatedly subject to cultural pressures for institutional care; pressures which persist to this day.

The historical origins and development of institutional care for people with learning difficulties

Burchinall (1982) pointed out that there is an inextricable link between the rise and development of institutional models of care for people with learning difficulties and prevailing social, cultural and political perceptions of them as a social group. Although life has probably always been tough for most disabled people, the process of industrialization and the rise of capitalism in the eighteenth and nineteenth centuries created new difficulties for them. The emphasis on a rationalized system of commodity production and social life can be seen to have created a new impetus for the provision of institutionalized 'care' for disabled people generally, including people with learning difficulties (Ryan and Thomas, 1987; Oliver, 1990). Like other groups of disabled people, people with learning difficulties found the newly industrialized and urbanized social environment, with its emphasis on time-keeping, productive efficiency and demanding physical labour, a hostile place in which to survive. People who may well have been able to contribute productively in an agrarian context where production was family based, governed by the hours of daylight and the rhythms of the agricultural year, risked becoming an unproductive economic burden on families reduced to living on subsistence wage labour. Added to this, a strong concern among commentators and policy makers in the taxpaying classes about the latent immorality of anyone who could not, or would not, work helped create the demand for a punitive, institutionalized system of control to be applied to the workless in all their variety. In Britain this approach was exemplified by the workhouse (Oliver, 1993b).

Elsewhere in Europe, rather more benign institutional forms of care were emerging. In France, for instance, in the early nineteenth century, the legacy of Revolutionary and Enlightenment thinking led to a more optimistic view of people with what we now term 'learning difficulties'. Seguin, for example, inspired by the educational work of his mentor Itard, and his *cause célèbre* 'Victor' the 'wild boy of Averyon', developed the idea of 'Asylums', as places of sanctuary where 'idiots' could be educated and trained to live and work in communities to which they would, ideally, be returned (Ryan and Thomas, 1987). In the UK, concern about the conditions inside institutions provided for 'idiots' also led to arguments for more benign regimes, such as that advocated by Tuke in York, who emphasized a regime of healthy work and strict morality (Dingwall et al., 1992). The late nineteenth century, however, saw a convergence of factors that led the institutions to adopt once more a custodial ethos.

The late Victorian era in Britain witnessed a confluence of moral and scientific authority, reflecting the pervasiveness of both the Protestant religion, bitterly divided at times between traditionalism and Nonconformism, and the political and economic self-confidence of a supremely self-assured political, economic and imperial elite. It was an era in which scientific knowledge and classification expanded exponentially, mainly in the service of imperial and economic expansion. It was an era too of grand scientific theorization. In 1859, for example, Charles Darwin published *The Origin of Species*. At the core of his thesis was the revolutionary idea that the evolution of species was driven, at least in part, by a process he called 'natural selection', the core argument being that in any species those individuals who are better able to adapt to the environment and conditions in which they find themselves – that is, are 'fittest' in survival terms – will be more likely to breed successfully and thus pass on the traits that made them successful. Conversely, those individuals less 'fit' in survival terms will be less likely to breed, and thus their lineages would fade away to extinction. Although in the *Origin* Darwin focussed on animal lineages to illustrate his theory, a number of his sympathizers quickly applied them to the analysis of human societies. It was Darwin's cousin Sir Francis Galton who went on to coin the term 'eugenics' to describe the application of Darwinian theory to human breeding (Desmond and Moore, 1991).

It was to both moral and scientific authority then that the members of the Eugenics Society appealed when making the case for action to prevent the 'degeneration' of national stock that they feared was imminent. Bolstered by a firm belief in their biological and social superiority, they saw themselves as responsible for the protection of the development of the race and society. Eugenic ideas were adopted across the political spectrum, with left-wing advocates using them to argue for birth control and family planning, whilst right-wing versions tended to emphasize the need for more coercive measures to stop undesirable elements, particularly 'feeble minded women', and, in the US, 'inferior races', breeding and swamping society with physically, mentally and morally degenerate progeny. Eugenic Societies on both sides of the Atlantic, and counterparts on the continent, came to dominate the social policy agenda on people with learning difficulties, or 'mental defectives' to use their terminology, in the late nineteenth and early twentieth centuries. Ideals of benevolence subsided as institutional regimes swung towards a custodial ethos (Kevles, 1985).

Despite the therapeutic rhetoric of psychiatry, a custodial and punitive ethos continued to dominate up to and beyond the nationalization of the large institutions with the inception of the National Health Service in 1947, when they were redesignated

'Mental Subnormality Hospitals'. In the 1960s and 1970s a growing revulsion at this situation came to a head with the exposure of a number of scandals involving brutality by nursing staff in various mental hospitals (Ryan and Thomas, 1987). The ensuing outcry led to official inquiries, and at the same time a number of influential studies appeared from both sides of the Atlantic which challenged the nature and purpose of institutional care for people with learning difficulties, regardless of whether they were subject to actual physical 'abuse' or not (Oswin, 1973; Bogdan and Taylor, 1976).

In 1971 the White Paper, *Better Services for the Mentally Handicapped*, was published: the first major review of service provision since 1929 (DHSS, 1971). National bodies were set up to lead change, with a significant role being played by psychologists rather than psychiatrists, reflecting the waning dominance of traditional medical psychiatry. The 1960s saw a growing influence of behavioural psychology. Based on the idea that people's behaviour is shaped by rewards and punishments contingent on them, behavioural psychology offered an explanation for the bizarre behaviours often demonstrated by people living in institutional environments, showing that many of them were self-stimulatory or learned, rather than inherent to their condition. It also suggested that if the environment and staff input were manipulated appropriately then people with learning difficulties could be taught, and could learn, appropriate, socially adaptive behaviours or skills, thus challenging the therapeutic pessimism that had so often dogged services (Gross, 1995). Although revolutionary in many ways, the influence of this new wave of psychological theory did not in itself challenge the institutional model of service provision. In fact, behavioural approaches were initially pioneered in hospital settings and were sometimes applied in ways that have since been decried as abusive (McGee et al., 1987). Emergent at the same time, 'normalization philosophy' did significantly challenge the structural and organizational nature of services.

Originating in Scandinavia, normalization philosophy was initially based on a human rights ethos, with pioneers like Bank-Mikkelson in Denmark, and Nirje in Sweden, arguing that large institutional environments were an affront to human rights and dignity. They advocated for service structures and practices approximating to that considered 'normal' for the particular society in which they were set (Emerson, 1992). It was in North America however, that normalization was elaborated into a more 'scientific' theoretical framework. Wolfensberger (1972) dropped the 'rights' emphasis of the Scandinavians, drawing heavily instead upon deviancy and labelling theory to explain the processes by which people with learning difficulties came to be devalued in society. He also used ideas such as 'role modelling', and the 'power of imitation', as useful tools for practice, and argued that the primary role of human services was to reverse the process of devaluation by enhancing the social image and competence of service users (Emerson, 1992).

For a time in the 1980s it appeared as though the 'normalization revolution' was actually happening, with community care policy leading to the closure of large institutions, and the people who had spent their whole lives in them experiencing the relative freedom of living in small group home environments. In reality, however, community care policy in the UK has been dominated from the outset by a fiscal agenda initiated by the 'new right' influenced Thatcher governments, rather than the emancipatory ethos of normalization philosophy. As the gloss has begun to wear off community care, so the realization has dawned that the two concepts of 'normalization' and 'community care' were by no means as synonymous as they may at one time have appeared.

Institutional care in the 'community care' era

As the shift towards community care continued, a growing body of research into the situation of people with learning difficulties living in community-based residential care developed. Much of this research has been concerned with gaining insight into their lived experience; a methodological lineage that can be traced back to the work of the pioneering American social scientist Erving Goffman and his analysis of the life of inmates in a large mental institution in the USA (Goffman, 1961). Goffman developed the concepts of the 'total institution' and the 'inmate world', and, although it is arguable that his concept of the 'total institution', a completely insular and isolated world where inmates live a life totally separated from wider society, was always an 'idealized' concept, it nonetheless highlighted the way in which institutions frequently became a 'world in themselves', with rituals, rules and roles that expressed a power above and beyond a therapeutic dynamic in relationships. Like that of Foucault (1977), Goffman's analysis highlighted the relationship between institutional practices and the exercise of disciplinary power, even where the regime was officially deemed to be therapeutic rather than punitive in purpose.

Subsequent research in community-based residential settings suggests that the concept of the 'inmate world' remains highly relevant in understanding the situation of people with learning difficulties. Humphreys, Evans and Todd (1987) for example, in a study of a community residential service in Cardiff, refer to people being drawn into the 'service world'. In a similar vein Sinson uses the term 'micro-institutionalization' to describe the situation she found in twelve group homes. She describes this as '[T]he transference of those institutional practices found in large-scale institutions to their small-scale community replacements' (1994: 267). Sinson's findings are bleak; she concludes that the people whose situation she explored experienced a dearth of 'subtle, self actualizing activity', that loneliness and isolation were common, and that a claustrophobic atmosphere of suffocating paternalism was pervasive. Sinson's conclusions are echoed in many other studies, including Malin (1983), Firth (1986) and Richardson and Richardson (1989). Much of this research was summarized by Emerson and Hatton (1994) who noted that, though community-based services undoubtedly marked an improvement on conditions in the large institutions, a picture nonetheless emerges of the persistent isolation of service users from mainstream society, a high degree of dependence on staff for meaningful relationships and activities, few opportunities to establish relationships beyond the 'service world', and the persistence of a divide between the 'service user world' and the 'staff world'. Similarly, Collins (1992), in a report that reviewed progress on the resettlement of people with learning difficulties into the community, noted the strong pressures to retain medicalized models of control and management of residents' lives. More recently still, Johnson and Traustadottir (2005) draw together accounts and research from around the developed world that suggest this is an issue by no means restricted to the UK.

The shift to community care can be characterized, therefore, as not so much a process of 'deinstitutionalization' as of 'reinstitutionalization'. People have been relocated from large isolated institutions into mini-institutions dispersed in the community. The lives that people lead are often still highly impoverished in comparison with the lives of comparable 'non-disabled' citizens. It is this situation that can be described as constituting 'institutional abuse', and its persistence continues to have serious detrimental consequences for the lives of people with learning difficulties. We can see this if we look specifically at the issue of the 'health' of people with learning difficulties; health being, it has been powerfully argued, the very foundation of well-being (Seedhouse, 2001).

Institutional abuse: the case of health

It is a major irony that, although for much of the last sixty years many people with learning difficulties have lived under the close surveillance of the NHS, they continue to suffer from a much higher incidence of health problems than most other sections of the population (Thompson and Pickering, 2001). Greenhaulgh (1994) examined some of the reasons for this, noting the undoubted impact of physiological factors associated with the cause of intellectual impairment itself, such as epilepsy, and that some conditions, or 'syndromes', are commonly related to particular health problems: heart defects, respiratory illness and dementia affecting people with Down's syndrome for example. Often, however, the health problems she identified were more general in nature, unrelated to the causation of intellectual impairment itself, but frequently going unreported or undetected. For example, problems with teeth, feet, hair, diet, weight and continence were all widespread in the studies reviewed by Greenhaulgh. Among the main reasons for this under-reporting and poor detection are problems with communication. Where an individual with learning difficulties has poor, or no, verbal communication they are reliant on care staff to pick up communicative behaviours that indicate a health problem, or a change in health status. For this to happen, care staff need to know the person well and be sensitive to idiosyncratic modes of communication.

For detection to occur care staff need also to have an awareness of health issues and problems that may affect the people they work with. The widespread move to dispersed social care, undertaken by private and voluntary sector organizations – often using untrained carers and high numbers of bank staff – that has resulted from the operation of community care policy has proven problematic in this respect. Greenhaulgh (1994) identified high staff turnover, frequent use of bank staff, lack of knowledge, awareness and training, and low expectations about the health of people with learning disabilities among care staff as important factors underlying the under-reporting and under-detection of common health problems. Thus highly restrictive levels of funding, consequent low wages, and relatively poor working conditions have resulted in a crisis in both numbers and in quality of staff in many services

Alongside this, research into the response of generic NHS services, on which people with learning disabilities have become more reliant as they have moved into the community, shows that a poor level of service is common (Hart, 2003). People with learning disabilities experience difficulty in accessing generic health care services, whether in hospital or in primary care, often as a result of ignorance, prejudice and poorly organized environments and organizations (Mencap, 1997; Carter, 2000). These deficits in health care, and the additional health problems faced by people with learning disabilities identified above, have led to a series of policy statements and guidelines from the Department of Health, the NHS Executive, and other governing bodies in the NHS and the health care professions, designed to improve performance in responding to the health needs of people with learning disabilities these include initiatives such as *The Patients Charter and You* (Hull and Holderness Community Health NHS Trust, 1995), 'The OK health check' (Mathews, 1997), *Feeling Poorly* (Dodd and Brunker, 1998), *Getting Better* (Band, 1997), and *The Healthy Way* (Department of Health, 1998) and culminate in the identification of 'health' as a major target area in the 2001 white paper *Valuing People* (Department of Health, 2001b). Targets set in that document include, as a matter of priority, widespread health screening for people with learning disabilities, and the designation of 'health facilitators' to manage this. This impact of these initiatives is still to be fully evaluated, but it is significant perhaps that some twenty years after the shift to community care the NHS is still struggling to respond appropriately to the basic health care needs of people with learning difficulties.

A major factor underlying this inadequate response is, somewhat paradoxically, a continuing tendency to pathologize disability in general and learning difficulties in particular. Poor physical and mental health in people with learning difficulties is too often seen, it appears, to be 'part of the condition' by many health professionals still steeped in the idea that disability equates with ill health, with the effect that actual health problems and issues faced by people with learning difficulties go unrecognized and unmet (Goble, 2000).

For much of the twentieth century the idea that disability was a purely biomedical phenomenon, equivalent in most respects to illness and thus in need of the same programmes of eradication and treatment applied to disease, went unquestioned. The growth of the independent living movement among physically disabled people in the USA and the UK in the 1970s and 1980s was associated, however, with the redefinition of the nature of disability. In the UK this was articulated by the Union of the Physically Impaired against Segregation (UPIAS) (Oliver, 1996). The UPIAS definition, widely adopted by the disability movement in the UK, opted for a dualistic definition in which 'impairment' is defined as the actual functional limitation experienced by the individual, whilst disability is redefined as the limitation imposed on people by a society which fails to recognize and organize itself to meet the needs of people with impairments. Disability becomes, therefore, a category of social oppression akin to gender and race (Oliver, 1996).

Key players in this oppression of disabled people have been, according to this critique, health and social care professionals who, it has been argued, have assumed power and control over the lives of disabled people in various ways, including by creating of bodies of knowledge and expertise about disability which are based, not on the lived experience of disabled people, but on objectivist, scientific discourses that start from negative assumptions of deficit, tragedy and abnormality. The practice of professions often reflects this, with disabled people deprived of control and influence over what happens to them, while their entire lives are held up for scrutiny as they are dehumanized to the status of 'cases' (Gillman et al., 1997).

It is in this way, it has been suggested by Nunkoosing (2000), that the lives of people with learning disabilities have become 'colonized' by 'expert' caring professions. McKnight (1978) advanced a similar argument, describing the effects of the way that the scientifically categorized problems experienced by individuals become 'encoded' into a language comprehensible only to the professional expert and the expert community to which they belong, a major effect of which is to mystify both the problem and its solution to the extent that client, or lay, evaluation becomes virtually impossible. It also means the potential for a dialogue with clients about service goals and outcomes is reduced to a level that does not threaten or challenge the dominance and authority of the professional expert. This applies especially where the location of the client's 'problem' is the mind itself, as is the case with people with learning disabilities. The mind/brain is seen in western culture as the seat of the autonomous self, personal individuality and, above all, of rationality. From this perspective, the self is characterized as self-contained, self-reliant, unique, separate, consistent and private (Wetherell and Maybin, 1997). To experience impairment of the mind/brain, then, is to be seen to lose all, or at least a critical part, of the self, and the consequent access to autonomy and independence that goes with it.

As a consequence people with learning difficulties are still often viewed with a 'professional gaze', to adapt a phrase from Foucault (1973), which constructs their identity, more or less unconsciously, according to the perspective of authoritative professional groups. The medium by which this construction occurs is authoritative, scientifically and politically legitimized discourse, which serves at the same time, as

Nunkoosing (2000) has pointed out, to invalidate the attempts of people with learning disabilities to name and speak their own lives and realities. Herein lies the root of the continued institutional abuse of people with learning difficulties, an abuse which compromises their very health and well-being; abuse not as random acts of criminality or violence, but as an integral part of the institutional systems upon which services are based.

Conclusion

Institutional models of care and support for people with learning difficulties are, as we have seen, inextricably linked with the role and identity of the caring professions. Abbott and Meerabeau (1998) have pointed out, however, that the term 'profession-alism' has multiple meanings. Professions are often looked at critically, but can also be viewed positively. For example, professionalism can be seen as a benchmark of perfor-mance, competence and moral quality. Friedson (1994) has argued that 'professional-ism' is itself an ideology, and that it naturally reflects the wider socio-cultural ideologies about the nature of professional competence, knowledge and morality. In Friedson's view, professions are, despite all the critiques, better than the alternatives, and are both necessary and desirable to maintain a 'decent' society.

A number of authors have advocated the development of new kinds of profession-alism which attempt to address and overcome the shortcomings of 'traditional' pater-nalistic forms of professionalism. Stacey (1992) argues for a 'new professionalism' focused on the ideal of service, rather than expertise and control. Other authors have argued that such a change requires a shift in the relationship between professionals and their clients. Davies (1995) advocates a new form of professionalism in nursing, built on constructing alliances with patients, clients and other health professionals via the medium of 'reflexive practice'. Likewise, Williams (1993) suggests a 'dialogue' based approach to the development of professional knowledge, drawing in particular from the experience of individual clients and client groups; a view that echoes the perspectives of both the disability movement and the self-advocacy movement for people with learning disabilities.

In my view, this is where the future of service provision for people with learning difficulties should lie. The social model of disability has provided us with a critique of professions and institutional practice that we cannot, and should not, ignore. Whilst the argument advanced by some (Davies, 1993) that professionals are purely 'parasitic' on disabled people is, I would contend, an overstatement, it is important nonetheless to recognize the extent to which their material interests are intertwined with the maintenance of the service systems and power structures within which they work, and to ensure that these pressures do not override the moral imperative to work in ways which contribute to the emancipation, rather than the oppression, of clients, both as individuals and as minority groups in society.

Leonard (1997) argues that the emancipatory project of the welfare state, the health and social care systems that partially comprise it, and the professions that inhabit it, can be rediscovered only by acknowledging the powerful role of discourse as a form of cultural production of identity and knowledge systems. In particular, there is a need to acknowledge and celebrate difference; a point emphasized also by 'social model of disability' theorists (Swain and French, 2000). A starting point, according to Leonard, is to refrain from pathologizing and homogenizing difference, a tendency deeply entrenched in the consciousness of many health professionals, whose impulse is often to objectify clients and conditions in line with powerful cultural imperatives to demonstrate an empirical foundation to their knowledge and practice. It is my view that – with a clear understanding that health is an 'aspect' of the lives of people with learning difficulties rather than a totalizing concept against which they and their very being should be perceived and measured – health professionals can potentially reshape their role to form part of an emancipatory and empowering project in the lives of the individuals they work with.

Practical examples of this kind of approach would include working with individuals with learning difficulties to construct joint narratives about their health, lives and social situations; an approach which helps them to name and claim their own experience, and which helps their carers and supporters to perceive them not merely as 'cases', but as 'subjects' with their own life stories, experiences, hopes and aspirations. Such work can have a transforming effect on professional consciousness and practice, fostering something approaching what McGee and Menolascino (1991) described as 'a psychology of interdependence'. The research referred to earlier by Gillman et al. (1997) is a good example of this kind of work in practice, as is the 'life-mapping' work of Gray and Ridden (1999), the dialogue-based work of Ramcharan (1997), and the case studies described in my own work relating to people with learning disabilities and challenging behaviours (Goble, 2000).

There are some promising signs, then, that these trends may lead to a more emancipatory and empowering role for health professionals in the lives of people with learning difficulties. History in this field should have taught us to take nothing for granted, however, and a commitment to the work of building alliances with people with learning difficulties must continue if the health professions are to function in the lives of their clients from a position of moral validity.

The Narratives of Disabled Survivors of Childhood Sexual Abuse

Martina Higgins

The substance of this chapter is based on a research project undertaken with seven disabled survivors of child sexual abuse who chose to share their stories of both intra-familial and extra-familial abuse (Higgins, 2006). My particular focus on child sexual abuse did not negate consideration of other important aspects of child abuse experienced by participants and common in such situations (Sullivan and Knutson, 2000). Nor did it detract from an evaluation of the abuses they witnessed of other disabled children, or the more generalized abuses/misuses of power experienced in differing organizational settings. The focus did, however, signify the need to raise awareness of a societal situation where disabled children are 3.14 times more likely to be sexually abused than their non-disabled peers (Sullivan and Knutson, 2000) and, despite this fact, research continues to marginalize this important issue (Westcott and Jones, 1999). My concentration on sexual abuse also intended to draw out the complex and, sometimes, contradictory relationship that exists for disabled survivors between child sexual abuse, the impaired body and identity formation (particularly sexual identity).

The chapter begins with consideration of the research process, which enabled the production of the narrative. It then considers the three major areas of concern that emerged from thematic data analysis – **power, identity** and **narrative**. With regard to the issue of power, the chapter explores the way in which a devaluing, impairment-related, societal discourse can affect how disabled children are treated within large organizations, and how these same attitudes can also infiltrate the functioning of some families. The following section on identity looks at how the combined impact of child sexual abuse and disability oppression disrupts identity formation and identity enactment in both childhood and later life. As becomes apparent in the final section, a disrupted identity formation also has implications for the individual's narrative production and their later battles to produce a more reflective and self-absolving narrative account of their experiences.

Facilitating narrative accounts

The sample for this study was acquired through a process of self-selection (Disch, 2001). Although it was acknowledged that this recruitment method would probably not produce a representative cross-section of the disabled population, this bias was felt to be preferable to the problems incurred when using a third party to explain one's research (Booth and Booth, 1997). The approach also determined that any potential respondent would have reached a significant stage in their personal healing process; enabling them to feel confident enough to 'speak out' and expose their realities. Advertising over a number of months produced seven suitable participants.

Ethical evaluation and re-evaluation played a critical part in the entire research process and formed the backbone of the research relationship. It determined that particular attention was paid to ensuring that participants had an adequate support system in place before sharing their story (Castor-Lewis, 1988). It also influenced personal practice principles and created a necessity to promote the active involvement of participants in the production of an accurate account of the self. I worked from the premise that the greater the control given to the participants, the less likely the research was to infringe their rights (Swain et al., 1998). Of particular concern was the potential for re-traumatization through involvement (Newman et al., 1997). This concern was countered, however, by the work of Disch (2001) who confirms that when participants are fully informed about the purpose of the research, and when they participate of their own free will, then they are able to manage the feelings the research generates and can use these feelings to further their own healing.

Narrative methodology was felt to be the most suitable method of capturing the depth and richness of participants' life stories. As narrative performance has been shown to take many forms (Ochs and Capps, 1996), a number of methods of narration were suggested to participants as a means of telling their story. Different methods were chosen by different participants and included material produced in face-to-face interviews, e-mail, poetry, story work and artwork.

Narratives of power

Participants' narratives demonstrate that the sexually abused disabled child is located at the collision point of a number of oppressive societal beliefs and practices. These oppressive attitudes impregnate the cultures of some organizations potentially reproducing themselves by the recruitment of like-minded employees and the creation of dysfunctional cultures (Salaman, 1979). The research demonstrates that the sanctioning of particular belief systems by an organization can lead to the creation of dubious professional practice, which sometimes involves the abuse of disabled children.

All of the participants had involvement with health care providers and the majority experienced a range of objectifying or dehumanizing practices: these involved the aggressive administration of drugs and procedures, and insensitivity to the trauma of surgery. In this following quote May talks about her experiences of medical consultations and the lack of ownership she felt for her own body. She further makes a linkage between this objectifying treatment and the potential for later sexual victimization:

> I also think that, like other disabled people, I lacked a sense of my own body belonging to me, and being private, of not having to be touched if I didn't want to be. This came from having to have many visits to the doctors and physiotherapists, and needing help to do things. I remember being paraded in front of doctors with very little on and feeling I was a thing for discussion rather than a person in my own right. This feeling got stronger as I got older. I was thirteen before I was given a choice about whether I kept appointments. When I exercised my choice by not going, then I was made to feel guilty by other professionals, which reinforced my feelings of 'what is the point?' This lack of a sense that your body belongs to you is an issue that non-disabled children do not have to face. And, again, I can't say that this makes us more of a target, but it does make us better victims as we are less likely to object or tell. (May)

Protracted periods of hospitalization, for Lizzie and Jean who also participated in the research, resulted in personal experience of sexual abuse, frequent incidents of physical abuse and the witnessing of the infanticide of another disabled child. Here, Jean talks about her experiences of physical abuse:

> So it would be in a bathroom, and I have the image of a very big steel bath, and tiles again, and she had a metal jug and it was very much like the kind of metal jugs that I remember at school that we used to have for juice. Exactly the same kind of jug that she would use, big and all dented. I would be sitting in this wide tub and she would be pouring water all over me, and also pushing me down. So

she would grab the back of my head and my chest and push me down into the
water. So I would be spluttering and trying to breathe, and not being able to
breathe. And again, all the sort of frenzied religious stuff was happening in what
she was saying to me: full of hate. Hatefulness was the thing that came across
so clearly to me. (Jean)

In relation to both Jean and Lizzie's experience, and sexual abuse occurring within an institution such as a hospital, Sullivan and Beech (2002) argue that any organization or institution where children are cared for is vulnerable to infiltration by paedophiles, both male and female. Despite the establishment of systems such as the Criminal Records Bureau, abusers still manage to slip through the net. Wardhaugh and Wilding (1993), who build on the work of Goffman (1961) and Martin (1984), broaden the analysis of institutional abuse of children from the exclusive focus on the individual psychopathology of the perpetrator to the consideration of organizational structures and processes which harbour practices such as physical and sexual abuse, and infanticide. They describe this phenomenon as the 'corruption of care' and cite a number of factors which play a significant part in the creation of abusive environments. This work supports the view that the institutionalization of disabled children needs to be kept to an absolute minimum.

Abuse/misuse of power was also experienced during participants' encounters with other organizations. Children who attended residential educational settings, spoke of inferior educational standards, controlling regimes and sexual abuse. In mainstream education, they encountered cultures where non-disabled children's taunts were left unchallenged by teaching staff, and uninformed teaching practices conspired to alienate disabled children further. Additionally, for Thomas and Lyn, who attended mainstream schools, child protection concerns were ignored or dealt with in an *ad hoc* fashion. There was clear neglect by the staff of the professional responsibility to communicate their concerns to the appropriate agencies. While it may be argued that some of these educational practices were symptomatic of that era, many can still be observed in current educational practice (Kenny, 2001; O'Toole et al., 1999; Davis and Watson, 2001).

Physical violence and sexual violation can be seen as just one manifestation of patriarchal power (Solomon, 1992), and are common in the families of both disabled and non-disabled children. In my study, and for some of the participants who experienced intra-familial abuse, society's devaluing assumptions relating to impairment were seen as infiltrating the functioning of the family and the behaviour of perpetrators. In Josh's case, as recognized in the work of other writers (Shakespeare et al., 1996), impairment, and the need for physiotherapy or help with intimate care tasks, created increased opportunity for sexually abusive incidents to occur:

Also, I remember after that when we were still in the same house where the toilet
and bathroom were downstairs, that occasionally I would mess myself and he

> *would use the opportunity of me having to have a bath, or having to clean me up, to abuse me. I was easily accessible; I was an easy target because of my disability. Because I had a disability, there was more opportunity to access me, and because I needed cleaning up in the bathroom, I was more available in the right places as well. (Josh)*

Oppressive attitudes to impairment were reflected in the general quality of parenting that some participants received. This influenced, amongst other things, their perception of themselves as 'burdens' or 'problems'. In the first quote below, May illustrates how being perceived as a 'problem' affected her ability later to disclose her sexual abuse. In the second quote, Lyn describes a complex set of emotions whereby being perceived as a problem later translated itself, in her mind, into feeling that she deserved to be sexually abused, or that being abused was one method of redeeming herself for being a problem:

> *I don't think that there was ever a chance that I would have told because of my feelings of having to make up for breaking up the family the first time round. For years I had been told I was an inconvenience, and that having someone with a disability in the house meant you couldn't do things. I was told that they couldn't have the holidays they wanted, they had to buy things they wouldn't buy normally, or replace things more often. These things just made me feel I was a nuisance, not good enough, and that I should support the family because I was costing them money. I came close to telling once or twice but just could not face the consequences of doing it. I thought my mother would hate me even more, and I thought I would lose contact with my youngest sibling who I am very close to. (May)*

> *The reverse of that is the feeling that you actually deserve it really. If anybody deserves it in the family you do. It's absorbing the problems. I used to have this fantasy that I was a sponge, and actually absorbing things like that (being sexually abused), becomes a good thing to do, it becomes your role. The many things that you can't do that other children can do in their families, like being musical, or if you are in a wheelchair being athletic, but you are able to do this! One thing that I did say to my therapist a while ago was that in all this time, between age 8 and age 14, although there was a sense in which I didn't acknowledge that there was anything wrong, I also knew that there was a girl at my school called Jeanette who everybody knew was being abused by her father. Everybody knew it, she was a wreck, and the awful thing is I can remember feeling contemptuous of her because she couldn't hack it, she couldn't handle it. (Lyn)*

The devaluation of disabled children is an issue prevalent in the writings of various authors (Ablon, 1990; Middleton, 1992; Thomas, 1998) and is an issue relevant to the involvement of health and social work practitioners supporting such families.

Middleton (1992) found tragedy discourse being nurtured at a very early stage by health professionals attending the birth of a disabled child. Thomas (1998), who investigated the issues from the perspective of the disabled child, found that her respondents told stories of parents who ranged from supportive allies to obstacles to psychological well-being. The features of her research, which were common to this study, included: fathers blaming mothers for their child's impairment, fathers resisting any physical contact with the disabled child, the child's fear of abandonment and the child's isolation.

One of the consequences of a process whereby a child is perceived as a burden is its impact on the parent–child attachment. Two participants in this study referred to problematic attachments, which were perceived to have different causes. May made the link between residential education and a poor parent–child bond. Chloe related a compromised attachment, where poor support systems were available to parents of children with hidden impairments. One of the major issues discussed by Bolen (2002) in her research, which bore some relevance to this study, was the behavioural manifestation of problematic attachments. Both Lyn and Chloe, who also experienced extra-familial abuse, made reference to their need, as children, to seek out attention from other adults outside the family home, the reasons for this behaviour stemming from differing sets of family dynamics. What also became apparent in my study was the contribution of a problematic attachment to the development of a distorted belief system; that is, the child coming to believe that she deserved to be sexually abused or that she had to compensate, in some way, for being a burden.

Narratives of identity

Disability oppression and child sexual abuse had a combined impact on participants' subsequent identity formation and identity enactment. It could be seen that a, sometimes fragile, sense of self, created by negative attitudes to impairment in early childhood was fragmented by the experience of child sexual abuse. This resulted in the creation of a series of dissociative behaviours and, for some, confused sexual identities that persisted into adulthood, affecting both their relationship with themselves and others. To illustrate the complexity of the situation I use a quote from Jean, who articulates the difficulties that sexually abused disabled children face when trying to forge an identity from an impossible starting position:

> One of the things that I discovered during my recovery was this idea about our physical bodies being a piece of evidence of ourselves and that when you're young, and possibly this carries on to some extent, where is the line between my self and my body/mind? If this person is saying to me my body is bad and evil then that's saying I'm evil. The big message that disabled children get, regardless of abuse, is that you are a problem, your body, therefore you, are a problem, a

disappointment, your impairment/difference or your 'self' has 'ruined' the idealized expectation of parenthood, and the perfect '10 fingers and toes' baby. I felt that very much, I felt the pain that my mother had about what was going on with my body and me, I was causing that pain and there was nothing I could do to change that. I think that disabled children get that message very clearly, and then when you are abused as well, and when the abuse is happening with your physical body, they all just get muddled up into this big knot, which can become huge self hate focused on the body, mind and self. (Jean)

No longer able to confidently inhabit their body, which now symbolized a site of conflict and confusion, children's emotional pain created by the sexual abuse experience was invariably internalized and found expression in either dissociative amnesia (forgetting), or the development of a range of self-destructive dissociative behaviours. These included anorexia, self-mutilation, substance abuse and suicide attempts. Dissociative behaviour is a common feature for children who are faced with an experience that is confusing and who have little control with regard to what is happening to their physical being (Provus McElroy, 1992; MacFie et al., 2001). Far from being pathological symptoms, these behaviours can be seen as constituting a logical expression of pain and confusion by a healthy child to an unhealthy (parental) environment (Summit, 1983). The hate and disregard for their body are confirmed by the actions of their perpetrators (Young, 1992). I would also argue that the need to dissociate and escape the body could be heightened for disabled children.

Despite this inherently disadvantaged starting position, participants spoke of a number of collective identities that they now own, some of which have provided a degree of self-validation and empowerment. Of particular significance is their identity as a survivor of child sexual abuse and the process that facilitated its acquisition. Participants used multiple and varying methods of reinterpreting their childhood experience to arrive at a place where they felt safe enough to 'break the silence' and identify as a survivor. For Thomas, the survivor identity is embraced wholeheartedly. For Jean, and symbolic of the progress made in her healing process (Phillips and Daniluk, 2004), the identity is now seen to be too limiting, potentially precluding other important aspects of the self. For Lyn, the process has been complicated by the potential for being burdened by another stigmatized identity, in addition to a disability identity (Vernon, 1999):

I'm the survivor. And that word … when my probation officer first used it, I laughed. I said, 'What do you mean I'm a survivor, I thought you only became a survivor if you went through Dachau, Belsen or Auschwitz, what's this survivor thing?' But she said, 'You are, you have come through your own holocaust, you've made it, you're a living witness to that and you've done that.' And I thought 'Christ yeah.' (Thomas)

Having said that, I also feel very much that I don't want this identity that is about being a survivor, I am much more than that, a lot of other things have happened in my life. (Jean)

You struggle so hard to be seen as a person and not just as a disability that you don't then want to add something that you also can be labelled with and no longer be seen as being you. You know an abuse case. It's quite subtle that, and I can feel that sort of drive in me. I just don't want to have another handy label stuck on, because that particular handy label, disability, has been there all the time and it takes such an effort to get people to see past the label. (Lyn)

In more problematic terms, child sexual abuse and disability interacted to negative effect as far as some participants' sexual identity was concerned. It created, for male participants, the difficulty of reconciling a same-sex encounter with a heterosexual identity. This finding also occurs in the research of others (Gilgun and Reiser, 1990; Durham, 2003), but in my study was complicated further, in Thomas's case, by his perpetrator telling him that he was enjoying the abuse experience. Equally, for female participants, there was also some disruption in their developing sexuality. May was preoccupied with producing cover stories in adolescence for any potential pregnancy. The asexual objectification of May, by her family, conflicted with a very real sexual experience that necessitated a requirement always to have a male friend/boyfriend in tow.

Later in life, some participants referred to the adverse affects of child sexual abuse on their ability to enjoy intimate sexual relationships, an issue commonly reported by non-disabled survivors of sexual abuse (Fromuth, 1986; Mullen et al., 1994; Fleming et al., 1999; Phillips and Daniluk, 2004). They reported interference in their ability to feel fully connected with their sexuality, and a general inability to trust potential partners. They also spoke of their involvement with violent and abusive men, a disruption of their intuitive responses that had led to a failure to identify dangerous situations, and re-experiencing episodes when involved in sexual acts. These re-experiencing episodes involved a psychological return to the abuse situation, which precipitated a need to remove themselves from the current encounter.

Narratives of the narrative

The process of storytelling, generally, requires a sense of the past (Plummer, 1995) and since most participants had spent significant periods of time psychologically 'not being there', the usual developmental process concerning narration of the self had become undermined. Later in life, when dissociative defences were less critical for survival, they were able to emotionally re-engage with the experience of child sexual abuse. This was either because an incident or circumstance triggered the recovery of a buried memory, or a life event drew, more solidly, the issue to the forefront of the mind.

For the two participants who had coped with the abuse by burying the memory, the recovered memory, although creating an increase in symptoms such as depression and anxiety (Elliot and Briere, 1995; Norman, 2000), also provided a meaning-making function for personality characteristics and past life events. Equally, for those who had partial or continuous recall, the reconnection with the experience had unpleasant manifestations and created a sense of narrative chaos (Frank, 1995):

> There was a constant feeling of not being able to not feel it anymore. I was apparently doing all right, I was still functioning at work, nobody was saying to me 'God what's wrong with you', so clearly I was still hacking it, and yet inside I felt awful. At its peak I was going 15 minute stretches of not thinking about killing myself. I was thinking 'If I can get through the next 15 minutes without thinking about it, and then the next one', and this was all without really consciously relating it to anything that had gone previously, I just felt dreadful. (Lyn)

Since it is felt by many academics that memories of life events are held in a narrative format (van der Kolk and van der Hart, 1991) and imparted through a process of storytelling, it seemed logical that storytelling should become the method employed by participants to re-establish a sense of narrative coherence. Therapy/counselling played a significant part in the recovery process for all but one participant. The therapeutic process was used to both confront their sense of entrapment in a self-deprecating belief system (Simon, 1998) and to substitute incompatible childhood stories for the correct story (Evans and Maines, 1995), which contained a narrative truth (Spence, 1982). Personal healing also involved an acknowledgement of the segments of the narrative that had been eroded, or, at the very least, severely tampered with. Some participants spoke of 'loss of childhood' and others referred to a 'loss of self'. Below Josh elaborates further on this loss of childhood and Jean comments on the lack of self:

> He stole my childhood and he stole it pretty early on. An introduction to sex and sexuality should happen naturally, it shouldn't happen at a forced pace, and I should not have been used as a rag doll. I should not have been used for someone else's pleasure at that age, and nobody should, and it took me a long time to get over it. (Josh)

> Abuse is obviously wrong for lots and lots of different reasons, but I think one of the things for me, about it, is it's like a kind of theft; a spiritual theft. (Jean)

Again, therapy was one avenue for acknowledging and mourning the losses experienced in childhood. For Lyn, the therapeutic encounter involved a re-parenting experience, and the 'acting out' of adolescence; a developmental period that had been denied because of the necessity to meet either the emotional or the sexual needs of her parents. Josh decided to use other imaginative methods such as a nurturing of his neglected 'child self' by an engagement in child-like pursuits such as the purchase of children's toys. Both Jean and Josh undertook additional reclaiming activities aimed at reinstating the self, such as the production of self-portraits, the use of mirrors, the repositioning, in a prominent place, of childhood photographs, and their involvement in the narrative research process.

The question of narrative credibility or reliability was an issue for several participants, particularly those who had recovered their memories from a prior state of amnesia. Although both Lizzie and Jean felt very confident about the validity of this recovered information, their narratives evoked variable reactions from family members. In Jean's case, she expressed scepticism about whether her narrative would be believed by the police and the legal profession. The generalized discrediting of recovered memory narrative is enmeshed with the recovered memory or false memory debate and symbolizes a societal backlash against the increased predominance of child sexual abuse narrative in the media (Campbell, 1988). This debate, however, is too complex for me to be able to offer a measured account of the opposing positions here. Nevertheless, feminism would view it as another means of dismissing the narratives of women (Saraga and MacLeod, 1997; Gaarder, 2000). In the context of this debate, disabled women such as Jean and Lizzie, whose discourse is subject to a general devaluation, have no choice but to state their recovered abuse narrative louder, clearer and with more veracity than non-disabled survivors.

Conclusion

This chapter illustrates how society, through processes of devaluation, places disabled children in situations of unacceptable risk. The weaving together of the combined experience of disability oppression and child sexual abuse has enabled the identification of key areas of a disabled survivor's life where difficulties later become greatly intensified. In that respect, the usual business of identity formation and narrative production, which is problematic for most non-disabled survivors of sexual abuse, becomes a more complex issue. Despite these difficulties, however, and through the clear articulation of their ever-evolving narrative, the participants in this study have demonstrated a determination to rise above their predicament and strive for a more autonomous mode of functioning. Their willingness and ability to 'speak out' about the experience of child sexual abuse represent, on a wider political level, the liberation of the voices of a previously silenced and devalued sector of society. It offers hope to other disabled survivors who are trying to find a voice, and reminds professionals of their duty to examine their organizational cultures and scrutinize their professional practices.

Section II

From A Different Viewpoint

6 Affirming Identity

John Swain and Sally French

For us, the editors, the notion of an affirmative model began with Sally's observation that while tragedy was the dominant view of impairment and disability, the writings of disabled people expressed a far more varied and positive picture. We have written and spoken about the possibilities of an affirmative model of disability and impairment on numerous occasions. The exploration of an affirmative model was part of our motivation for producing this edited book. It is a way of thinking that directly challenges presumptions about the experiences, lifestyles and identities of people with impairments. Throughout history and in most cultures disabled people have been viewed as inferior, dangerous, tragic, pathetic and not quite human. Such are the negative presumptions held about impairment and disability, that the abortion of impaired foetuses is barely challenged (Parens and Asch, 2000a) and compulsory sterilization of people with learning difficulties was once widely practised in many parts of the world (Park and Radford, 1999). In 1986 Oliver wrote:

> It has to be remembered however, that personal tragedy theory itself has performed a particular ideological function of its own. Like deficit theory as an explanation of poor educational achievement, like sickness as an explanation of criminal behaviour, like character weakness as an explanation of poverty and unemployment, and like other victim-blaming theories (Ryan, 1971), personal tragedy theory has served to individualise the problems of disability and hence to leave social and economic structures untouched. (1986: 16)

Affirmation is expressed through resilience and resistance to the dominant personal tragedy model.

There are dangers that we shall recognize here and return to in the conclusion to this chapter. The first is in relation to disability, or more particularly the

(Continued)

(Continued)

social model of disability. The following statement from UPIAS, an organization of disabled people instrumental in establishing the social model of disability, addresses disability as political, a form of oppression.

> *We are oppressed by the society in which we live. How can there be 'advantages' out of this condition? It is true that all societies have hitherto oppressed their physically impaired citizens. Some will argue that this is intrinsic to physical impairment. We must insist, however, that the argument is about Britain today and that we are struggling against this oppression irrespective of whether it has always occurred. (1972: 7)*

If there are no advantages in being disabled, then an affirmative model of disability seems at best questionable and at worst justifying the status quo.

The second danger is in relation to impairment. The social model of disability has been subjected to criticism on a number of grounds, which have planted the seeds of controversial and dynamic debates. As Oliver (2004) points out, the first of these is that the social model, supposedly, ignores personal experiences of impairment, such as physical pain. For instance, research with people with high spinal cord injuries found that the physical manifestations of their impairments were of central concern to the participants: 'because sometimes you just can't get out of bed: you may have a pressure sore or not be feeling well ... it's not as easy as an able-bodied person' (Hammell, 1998: 76). Thus, on similar grounds, affirmation may be thought to be denial of the daily realities and experiences of being impaired, or as being brave in the face of tragedy. (Tragic But Brave was the title of an arts review organized and presented by disabled artists that toured the UK in the 1990s; a website; and a song – see pp. 73–74 below.)

A third possible line of critique focuses on the notion of identity. Basically, the affirmation of a disabled identity can be seen as, at the very least, over-simplistic and questionable in a number of ways (Ferguson, 2003). No disabled person is solely disabled: they are young, old, working-class, upper-class, male, female, gay, lesbian, heterosexual, Black, white, Asian, Christian, Muslim, atheist – and so on. The picture becomes complicated further if impairment is seen as an important factor defining identity: dividing people by type of impairment, age of onset, severity of impairment and so on. Critiquing the 'identity model', Fraser, for instance, could be writing about the affirmation of a disabled identity:

> *The overall effect is to impose a single, drastically simplified group-identity which denies the complexity of people's lives, the multiplicity of their identifications and the crosspull of their various affiliations. (2000: 112)*

In this chapter we explore these issues by focusing first on the general notion of identity and associated concepts of culture. We shall then turn specifically to the affirmation of disabled identity as both a personal and a political process which may be enacted and expressed in numerous ways. To conclude, we shall return to the lines of criticism outlined in this introduction.

Identity and culture: the personal and the political

Identity is the way people view themselves, how they view themselves in relation to others, and how they are viewed by others. It allows us to address seemingly straightforward questions: Who am I? and Who are you? As is typical in the social sciences, however, the seemingly simple becomes complex, with quite diverse viewpoints taken within different theoretical perspectives. Nevertheless, there are some key ideas within the umbrella notion of identity.

- It involves active engagement, individual and/or collectively, in the continual processes of identity formation and maintenance.
- In affirmation of identity the personal becomes social/political and the political becomes personal.
- Identity involves shared identification with some people and not others, through a myriad of social interactions, symbols and meanings.
- It also involves a tension between the control the individual has in constructing his or her identity and the social constraints limiting and determining identity formation.

Throughout this notion of identity then is a sense of 'us' and 'them'. Identity and social division or difference are closely interconnected issues and have increasingly come to prominence in areas of inquiry across the social sciences (Hetherington, 1998). Our sense of who we are, our own identity in relation to (sometimes versus) the identity of others, are part and parcel of our lived experience and interwoven, and created within, our interactions with others. Our sense of who we are is linked, for instance, to our awareness of our identities as women or as men. Both gender and sexuality can play a significant role in our understanding of identity, but, of course, what it means to be a man or woman, heterosexual or gay also depends on the society we live in. Identity is at the interface between the personal, that is thoughts, feelings, personal histories, and the social, that is the societies in which we live and the social, cultural and economic factors which shape experience and make it possible for people to take up some identities and render others inaccessible or impossible (Woodward, 2000).

Politics of difference can divide society into opposing groups, into 'them and us' and 'self and other', and where there is difference there is the potential for institutionalized discrimination: that is the unfair or unequal treatment of individuals or groups which is built into institutional organizations, policies and practices at personal, environmental and structural levels. Thompson (2001: 140) suggests that forms of oppression can impact on identity in a number of ways:

- alienation, isolation and marginalization – social exclusion from full participation in society;
- economic position and life-chances;
- confidence, self-esteem and aspirations; and
- social aspirations, career opportunities and so on.

Turning to disabled people and the formation of disabled identity, clearly there are social, cultural and economic factors that can have an impact (Priestley, 2003). Exclusion, the denial of the rights and responsibilities of citizenship and oppression shape experiences, expectations and personal and collective identities in many ways. Young identifies women, gays and lesbians, indigenous populations and disabled people as 'marginalized identities'. She argues, too, that marginalized groups 'are not oppressed to the same extent or in the same ways' (1990: 40). There are numerous specific examples of the oppression of disabled people in the chapters in Section I, particularly as manifestations of the personal tragedy model of disability.

It is only possible here to indicate some of the factors that may impinge on the identities of disabled people. Perhaps the most readily recognised are the barriers to access and participation. As Priestley states:

> Barriers to participation in the socially valued labour of production and reproduction have denied many disabled people access to the social networks and citizenship rights upon which autonomous adult identities are premised. (2003: 192)

Another general factor is the dominant individual, particularly medical, model in defining disability and underpinning ostensible treatment and rehabilitation. For instance, the continuing perceived imperative for the prevention of impairment using antenatal screening and abortion and the development of genetic technologies for the eradication or 'cure' of impairments devalues disabled people and their lives. The accompanying debates are rarely informed by the voices of disabled people themselves, though the possible impact on disabled identities is clear.

The third general factor is the images of disability in the mass media – or, more generally, cultural texts. The impact of media on our constructions of selves and others' identities can be profound and can lock people into ways of interacting which perpetuate the status quo and reinforce identities that individuals may not choose for themselves. As Gleeson (1999) suggests, the reductive stereotypes of disabled people – as dependent, abnormal (or freakish), helpless, or heroic and brave (in the face of tragedy) – limit the identities accessible to disabled people (including sexual, gendered and ethnic identities).

Affirmation: I am who I am

Within the confines of the social context, we actively and continuously negotiate who we are with those around us, in social interaction. It is fluid and changing. Concern about identity is concern about change: challenging social expectations about identity; establishing new identities; and transforming existing identities (Jenkins, 1996). This is collective as well as personal/individual. Since the 1950s 'new social movements', including the women's movement, the Black Power movement and the disabled people's movement, have played a significant role in the politics of identity. They can be seen as collective endeavours to give voice to and affirm new identities. It is apparent that the more overt the discrimination and oppression that people experience, the more heightened their awareness and sense of vulnerability will be around that particular identity. Monks states:

> People who are socially excluded and oppressed, and who are often also defined as lacking qualities of a normative social being, may find solidarity in the shared experience of exclusion itself ... The 'communities' which emerge may become politically active ... Experience of the interdependence, mutuality and solidarity which arise from shared activities and communication is an important part of membership, even of direct political action. (1999: 71)

Similarly, Hetherington suggests that identity has become significant through resistance to dominance in unequal power relations:

> One of the main issues behind this interest in identity and in identity politics more generally has been the relationship between marginalisation and a politics of resistance, and affirmative, empowering choices of identity and a politics of difference. (1998: 21)

Questions of identity, then, take analysis into the collective political arena. Jenkins writes of resistance as potent affirmation of group identity:

> Struggles for a different allocation of resources and resistance to categorisation are one and the same thing ... Whether or not there is an explicit call to arms in these terms, something that can be called self-assertion – or 'human spirit' – is at the core of resistance to domination ... It is as intrinsic, and as necessary, to that social life as the socialising tyranny of categorisation. (1996: 175)

By moving to a position of viewing disability as both a personal and a public or political issue, the disabled person becomes empowered to confront the cultural stereotypes, discrimination and environmental barriers that undermine quality of life and identity (Swain and Cameron, 1999).

It is our contention that an affirmative model is developing out of individual and collective experiences of disabled people that directly confronts the personal tragedy model not only of disability but also of impairment. The notion of affirmation is one of great depth – taking us into what we are as human beings. From the documented viewpoint of disabled people, far from being tragic, being disabled can have benefits. There are numerous ways in which disabled people are affirmative that we can only touch upon.

1   Perhaps at the most basic level, impairment is simply a 'fact of life'. A participant in Watson's research typifies this:

> Tommy argued that 'I don't wake up and look at my wheelchair and think "shit, I've got to spend another day in that", I just get up and get on with it'. (2002: 519)

Kent writes:

> I will always believe that blindness is a neutral trait, neither to be prized nor shunned. (2000: 62)

2   Affirmation can be of self, 'I am what I am', in direct opposition to the tragedy view of being disabled. The following quotation from Phillipe, a participant in a research project, turns the tragedy model on its head. The tragedy would be to be cured of impairment rather than being impaired:

> I just can't imagine becoming hearing, I'd need a psychiatrist, I'd need a speech therapist, I'd need some new friends, I'd lose all my old friends, I'd lose my job. I wouldn't be here lecturing. It really hits hearing people that a deaf person doesn't want to become hearing. I am what I am! (in Shakespeare et al., 1996: 184)

The next quotation is taken from the work of a disabled person produced in a workshop run by a disability arts organization. This poem is about the rejection of shame, or tragedy, to be countered by pride engendered by collective affirmation of disabled identity.

Sub Rosa

Fighting to establish self-respect...

Not the same, but different...

Not normal, but disabled...

Who wants to be normal anyway?

Not ashamed, with heads hanging,
Avoiding the constant gaze of those who assume
that sameness is something to be desired...
Nor victims
of other people's lack of imagination...
But proud and privileged to be who we are...
Exactly as we are. (Tyneside Disability Arts, 1998)

3   Affirmation can be of self in the face of the discrimination/oppression faced by disabled people, challenging social norms that set or carry expectations and also the personal devaluation when norms are not met.

I do not wish for a cure to Asperger's Syndrome. What I wish for is a cure for the common ill that pervades too many lives, the ill that makes people compare themselves to a normal that is measured in terms of perfect and absolute standards, most of which are impossible for anyone to reach. (Holliday Willey, 1999: 96)

A disabled man quoted by Shakespeare et al. said, 'I am never going to be able to conform to society's requirements and I am thrilled because I am blissfully released from all that crap. That's the liberation of disfigurement' (1996: 81).

4   Some disabled people affirm their lifestyle/quality of life as against the presumed tragedy of lack or loss of lifestyle/quality of life. Becoming impaired is not necessarily experienced as a loss or deterioration. For some it is a far-reaching life change that can be negotiated in different ways. A woman quoted by Morris states:

As a result of becoming paralysed life has changed completely. Before my accident it seemed as if I was set to spend the rest of my life as a religious sister, but I was not solemnly professed so was not accepted back into the order. Instead I am now very happily married with a home of my own. (1989: 120)

People born disabled may also feel that being disabled has contributed positively to the lifestyles they have established and led. For Vasey, disability opened rather than closed possibilities for personal relationships:

We are not usually snapped up in the flower of youth for our domestic and child rearing skills, or for our decorative value, so we do not have to spend years disentangling ourselves from wearisome relationships as is the case with many non-disabled women. (1992: 74)

For Tom, impaired by the drug thalidomide, being disabled provided a context in which he created opportunities and choices:

> Life is very good ... being born with no arms has opened up so many different things that I would never have done. My motto is 'In life try everything'. I wouldn't have that philosophy if I'd been born with arms. (Archive Hour BBC Radio 1, June 2002)

5   Disabled people collectively affirm self and disabled identity in their struggle against discrimination and oppression. The notion of disability culture and disability arts is important here. Peters (2000) identifies two views of culture that are particularly relevant to understanding the affirmation of identity. The first she calls social/political. This is the collective voice of disabled people grounded in a common goal, but with 'multiple expressions, pathways, needs' (2000: 590). She states:

> As Shakespeare notes: 'In making "personal troubles" into "public issues" disabled people affirm the validity and importance of their own identity. (2000: 501)

Another view of culture is as personal/aesthetic. Peters writes:

> For those who subscribe to the view of culture as personal/aesthetic, the ability to assert an aesthetic pride in the disabled body is a necessary prerequisite to political identity and is the source of empowerment. (2000: 592)

The following two quotations were generated through the work of a disability arts group. They seem to speak to both the social/political and personal/aesthetic views of disability culture.

> We are who we are as people with impairments, and might actually feel comfortable with our lives if it wasn't for all those interfering busybodies who feel that it is their responsibility to feel sorry for us, or to find cures for us, or to manage our lives for us, or to harry us in order to make us something we are not, i.e. 'normal'. (Tyneside Disability Arts, 1999: 35)

Coming Out

> And with the passing of time
> you realise you need to find
> people with whom you can share.

There's no need to despair.

Your life can be your own

and there's no reason to condone

what passes for their care.

So, I'm coming out.

I've had enough

of passing and playing their game.

I'll hold my head up high.

I'm done with sighs

and shame. (Tyneside Disability Arts, 1999: 35)

We end this section with extracts from the lyrics of a song that is well known to disabled activists. It expresses some if not all of the ways of affirming disabled identity summarized above. It does so with wit and irony, lampooning that defining image of disability in the dominant western culture, tragic but brave.

Tragic But Brave
(by Mike Higgins and Ian Stanton)

Just a way to ease the boredom

Propaganda all around

He swallows all the spiel he's given

Deliverance so easily found

He smiles for the cameras

Never wears a frown

Until the lights go down

Because he's tragic but brave

And he knows that Jesus saves

He could be whole

If he could just hold God's hand

You know he's tragic but brave

And oh so well behaved

And he knows it's all a part

of God's eternal plan

'Cos he's a sinful man.

Beads of sweat and muscles straining

Supercrip's the way she'll stay

So she can be a human being

Not disabled in any way

Someone will always help her

Up the steps at work each day

Hide it all away.

He stumbles down the street with shopping

All the people smile his way

What it is to be independent

He will gladly hear them say.

He falls through the front door

And rubs the pain away

It's just a part of his day.

And he looks at the crowd on the TV news

With their wheelchairs, their sticks and their guides

They are brandishing banners

They are pissing on pity

And they celebrate difference with pride

Something stirs inside.

Something moves inside

Something recognises...

Something stirs inside.

Conclusion

The affirmative model directly challenges presumptions of personal tragedy and the determination of identity by the value-laden assumptions of non-disabled people. It signifies the rejection of dominant social beliefs about disabled people and their lives, alongside rejections of notions of dependency and abnormality. Whereas the social model is generated by disabled people's experiences in a disabling society, the affirmative model is born of disabled people's experiences as valid individuals, as determining their own lifestyles, culture and identity. It is certainly not a model of disabled people's identity or lives, as they are, can or should be. It is fundamentally about critique, the critique of supposed tragedy. It challenges the images and discourses of disability and impairment that convey and construct people and their lives as by necessity tragic. The affirmative model is, thus, not a model for judging disabled people's feelings and understandings of themselves and their lifestyles/quality of life (whether or not they have recently acquired an impairment) but it is a model that stands in opposition to the dominant, 'commonsense' beliefs about disabled people's feelings about themselves, their bodies and their lives. The social model says that all disabled people are subjected to discrimination/oppression, whether or not they feel or understand themselves to be. The affirmative model says that all disabled people are subjected to a tragedy view of themselves and their lives, whether or not they feel or understand themselves to be subjected to such a view.

In this light we shall return to and review the possible critiques of an affirmation model raised in the introduction to this chapter. First, disabled people do affirm lifestyles despite the oppression and discrimination they may experience on a daily basis. This can indeed be interpreted as passivity and compliance but this seems to us to miss the underlying political message, which is that inclusion, or mainstreaming, can only be effective if it is on disabled people's terms. It is not a matter of accepting non-disabled people's norms, or normal identities. In affirming different lifestyles disabled people provide the counter-narrative to the dominant narrative of non-disabled people. It is from such experiences that disabled people can look, for instance, for 'the reconfiguration of work for disabled people' (Barnes and Roulstone, 2005).

The second possible criticism is that the affirming of disabled identity denies daily experience of impairment. As Barnes and Mercer state:

> the 'celebration of difference' is problematic for many disabled people, particularly those whose impairments are debilitating, painful or perhaps associated with premature death. (2003: 77)

Though we have collected many expressions affirming disabled identity over the years, only a few of which are included in this chapter, it would be nonsense to claim that all disabled people make positive affirmations of their identity. Indeed, such a claim could not be made about any group: women, Black people, children. This is not the claim of an affirmative model and such a criticism is based on a conceptual misunderstanding. The affirmative model is a direct challenge to the personal tragedy model. Though people whose impairments are debilitating, painful or associated with premature death *may* find affirmation problematic, the real problem is the assumption that they will necessarily, simply because of being impaired, experience their lives and

themselves as personal tragedies, to the extent that it would have been better not to
have been born.

The third line of possible criticism is that identities are fractured, fluid, multiple and
contested. We are all a complex amalgam of multiple aspects of identity and members of
several different socially divided groups. Social divisions are not simply additive either in
terms of disadvantage or identity. Black disabled women, for instance, experience forms of
discrimination that can connect and overlap and reinforce each other, in being Black and
disabled and female. Membership of different socially divided groups can operate in contradictory and complex ways (Vernon and Swain, 2002).

Such views are important in relation to the affirmation of disabled identity. Affirmation
of identity is a continuing process rather than an end product: there is no essential disabled
identity. Indeed, the affirmation of disabled identity is generated, at least in part, by the disavowal of the limited, the status quo, stereotypes, the typecast, the predetermined. Barnes
and Mercer make a similar point with reference to disabled identity:

> The designation of an individual as a 'disabled' person does not result in a fixed
> identity, but should be thought of as a narrative that is constantly being reworked
> or 'retold'. (2003: 79)

It is nonsensical to conceive of a society that is inclusive of disabled people but is
racist, sexist, ageist or homophobic. Similarly it seems to us to be nonsense to affirm
disabled identity through the denial of sexual, ethnic or other identity. Thomas (1999)
comes to a similar conclusion. She promotes a 'narrative identity' approach, which
centres on the stories we tell of ourselves, 'the storied quality of self-identity', within
the context of 'public narratives', basically the stories (media images and so on) surrounding disabled people. She recognizes the social model, generated by the disabled
people's movement, as providing a counter-narrative to the dominant stories of the
individual, particularly medical, models. Similarly we would argue that the affirmative
model is a counter-narrative to the prejudices, expectations, actions and practices
predicated on a personal tragedy model of disability. Thomas goes on to state:

> Other counter-narratives which contest the public narratives of gender, 'race',
> sexuality, age and so on are also of critical importance to the many disabled
> people who are marginalized in other ways – because they are women, black,
> gay, older and so on. These make up other elements of their self-identities, but
> they do not exist in separate psychic departments and so cannot be seen as
> outside, or nothing to do with, disability politics. On the contrary, they suffuse
> and thus enrich disability politics: 'Oppressed people resist by identifying
> themselves as subjects, by defining their reality, shaping their new identity,
> naming their history, telling their story' (bell hooks, cited in Plummer 1995: 30).
> (1999: 120)

Some Key Questions to Address in Section 2

Activity

Collect examples of visual art, poetry, autobiographical statements and narratives by disabled people. Twenty years ago this would have been a difficult activity as there was little of this material to be found. There is now a plethora of examples, as you will find from even a cursory search of the literature and the internet. The only criterion for selecting your examples is that they are produced by disabled people themselves. With each example reflect on the messages being created by disabled people about disability, impairment and their lives. This activity forms an excellent basis for a group discussion with colleagues or fellow students.

Questions

The chapters in this section explore the experiences of disability and impairment as expressed by disabled people themselves. As you read spend some time thinking, and if possible discussing, your reactions to this. You might find it helpful to consider the following.

1   An affirmative model of disability and impairment challenges the presumptions of the tragedy model. List ways in which such challenges can be expressed.
2   The affirmative model is founded in the social model of disability. There is wide acknowledgement by disabled people of the power of the social model in analysing, critiquing and challenging the oppression of disabled people and in changing disabled people's lives. In this context what does the affirmative model offer in disabled people's struggles for full participative citizenship?
3   The affirmative model draws on the personal experience of disabled people and addresses notions of impairment as well as disability. What are the dangers of furthering an individual model – that 'the problem' lies within the individual? How does an affirmative model challenge an individual model?
4   The chapters in this section address the affirmation of disabled people and their lives as disabled. No disabled person's identity is solely as disabled. Disabled people's identities, like those of non-disabled people, incorporate

(Continued)

(Continued)

gender, age, ethnicity, impairment and sexuality. It is possible, for instance, to affirm personal identity as both a visually impaired and a disabled person. As you read the chapters in this section consider the implications for the celebration of difference across all social divisions.

5   As in the previous section, critically reflect on your personal understandings of disability and impairment. A question for both non-disabled and disabled people is: how far can non-disabled people understand and empathize with the experiences and views of disabled people, particularly when they contradict strongly held presumptions?

Choices, Rights and Cabaret: Disability Arts and Collective Identity

Allan Sutherland

The movement that we describe as 'disability arts' has developed over the last three decades, as disabled people have rejected negative assumptions about their lives, defined their own identities, expressed pride in a common disabled identity and worked together to create work that reflects the individual and collective experience of being disabled.

Disability arts antecedents

There have always, of course, been great artists with impairments. These are not forgotten figures; this is not the same issue as that which occurs in women's art, where feminist art historians have laboured to research the careers of women artists whose achievements had been sidelined, uncovering work that has been unjustly forgotten about. Many of the most famous names in the western cultural canon have been known as disabled people, including Homer, Milton, Goya, Pope, Beethoven and Vincent van Gogh. (I am aware that these figures are all male, and would refer my readers to the feminist discourses cited above for the reasons. The general principle holds in the case of such lesser figures as Elizabeth Barrett Browning, Dorothea Lange and Frida Kahlo.)

The examples I have cited are all figures who are publicly known to have been disabled, to the extent, in some cases, that the impairment has become part of the popular mythology surrounding the artist. (In Homer's case, it may be nothing *but* mythology; the poet is reputed to have been a blind wandering minstrel, but the actual facts of his life are little known.)

Such myth-making easily leads to misreadings of the work. It is attractive, for example, to look at the frenetic swirling skies of a Van Gogh landscape and see them as outpourings of the artist's inner turmoil. (Van Gogh, the archetypal tortured genius, is perhaps *the* most mythologized of artists in this way.) Examination of the artist's earlier work, however, shows that he developed this style as a result of painstaking analysis of Japanese styles of decoration.

These artists did not, on the whole, treat their own disabilities as suitable subjects for their work. There are exceptions to this rule. One of the best known is Milton's sonnet 'On His Blindness', where the poet wrestles with the question of how to serve God now that he has lost his sight, arriving at the conclusion that to bear his situation with stoicism is itself a service:

> God doth not need
>
> Either man's work or his own gifts; who best
>
> Bear his milde yoak, they serve him best, his state
>
> Is kingly: thousands at his bidding speed
>
> And post o'er land and ocean without rest;
>
> They also serve who only stand and wait. (Milton, 2003: 81)

Milton was a great poet, but he's a non-starter as a role model for other disabled people.

A less acquiescent approach can be found in the work of Alexander Pope, who describes being at the mercy of sycophants who tried to win him over with flattering responses to his impairment. Only a dunce would patronize someone of Pope's sharp wit, but fashionable society, then as now, was full of dunces:

> There are who to my person pay their court:
>
> I cough like Horace, and, though lean, am short
>
> Ammon's great son one shoulder had too high –
>
> Such Ovid's nose – and 'Sir, you have an eye'.

The great satirist gave such approaches short shrift, responding to them with a devastating dismissal:

> Go on, obliging creatures, make me see
>
> All that disgraced my betters met in me.
>
> Say, for my comfort, languishing in bed,

'Just so immortal Maro held his head;'

And, when I die, be sure and let me know

Great Homer died three thousand years ago. (Pope, 1961: 10)

What such poems have in common is solitude. They are both poems that treat disability as something contained in the individual, a cross the poet has to bear. (Shortly after the passage quoted above, Pope refers to 'this long disease, my life'.)

A particularly interesting example, to my mind, occurs in a poem that is not generally thought of as being about disability or impairment: Edward Lear's 'nonsense' poem, 'The Pobble who has no Toes'. The Pobble, one of Lear's happier characters, is warned that he may lose his toes by the disapproving 'they', who provide a regular chorus to Lear's poems, but he refuses to be downhearted:

When they said, 'Some day you may lose them all;'

He replied – 'Fish fiddle de-dee!'

Following advice, he carries out preventative measures such as drinking 'lavender water tinged with pink' and wrapping his nose in scarlet flannel. But when he sets out to swim the Bristol Channel, a passing porpoise takes the flannel and he subsequently finds that his toes have gone. But the poem finishes with the optimistic words of his steadfast ally, Aunt Jobiska:

'It's a fact the whole world knows,
'That Pobbles are happier without their toes.' (Noakes, 2001: 397–398)

Read as a poem about disability written by a disabled man (Lear struggled all his life with epilepsy and depression), it yields a surprisingly modern meaning for disabled people: a disabled identity is more fulfilling than a fruitless attempt to be a second-rate able-bodied person.

This is a valid conclusion, whose practical application can be seen, for example, in what happened in the wake of the thalidomide affair. As the 'thalidomide babies' matured into thalidomide toddlers, they were presented with a range of elaborate prosthetic arms and legs. Without exception, they rejected them.

I do not think I am merely imposing this meaning on the poem. It's not even a difficult message to see, at least for a disabled person. So why is this usually treated as a nonsense verse, a children's poem? My suspicion is that positive messages about disability are simply so unfamiliar in our culture that they just don't get recognized.

Disability arts has its antecedents in the visual arts as well. Consider, for example, Van Gogh's self-portraits of himself with a bandaged ear. As he had severed his own earlobe during a mental crisis, it was undoubtedly a courageous act to make public reference to the episode. (Such must have been his decision; he could easily have painted himself facing in the other direction, as he did on various other occasions.) I doubt very much, however, if the decision in any way represented a gesture of solidarity with other disabled people, which would be the case for an artist working within disability arts.

The Mexican painter Frida Kahlo depicted her impairment in a number of works, the most significant being *The Broken Column*. The artist stands erect in front of an empty landscape (a common surrealist feature), naked from the waist upwards, her torso encircled tightly by bands of leather or metal. Her chest is cut open like an anatomical illustration to reveal her spine, which is depicted as a broken Ionic column. All over her body, her skin is pierced by nails – presumably a metaphor for her constant physical pain, but also a clear reference to Christian iconography.

Opinions vary as to the significance of Kahlo's representation of her own disability. It is interesting to find such strong portrayals of a personal experience of disability, but it is questionable whether she is moving away from a tragedy model. Liz Crow, director of the short film Frida Kahlo's Corset (http://www.roaring-girl.com/), refers to her as 'a drama queen' (personal communication). Michael Shamash, reviewing the Tate Modern's exhibition of Kahlo's work in *Disability Now*, described her as iconic, but not a good artist: 'Frida is fascinating in her promotion of the artist as celebrity. She also was important in expressing impairment in art. Her most interesting creation was the myth of Frida Kahlo. She was the Tracey Emin of her day' (Shamash, 2005).

Pioneering disability arts

These are all interesting and significant precursors, but they are not disability arts. Consider the difference between the earlier poems and 'Scars' by the late Simon Brisenden, one of the pioneers of Independent Living in the UK, an important activist and theorist:

> The man who cut your skin
> and delved within
> has he got any scars?
>
> the man whose sterile slice
> left mind and body in a vice
> has he got any scars?
>
> the man who bent your bones
> and organised your personal zones
> has he got any scars?
>
> the man who laid you flat
> and said I'm in charge of that
> has he got any scars?

> *you do not cry alone*
>
> *in rage*
>
> *his blood is on this page. (Brisenden, C. 1987: 8)*

Several things make this poem different in quality to the work described above. For a start, it works consciously within the social model of disability, and is empowered by it. The whole poem is infused with righteous anger, based on the presumption that *things do not have to be like this*. Milton's blindness may have been an unavoidable fact, but the behaviour of arrogant surgeons is not.

The poem is therefore about much more than just what has happened to one person. It is about how disabled people get treated in a discriminatory society, about sexism ('the *man* who cut your skin'), medical paternalism and the imbalance of power that allows disabled people to be treated like this, with no choice in the matter. It is also implicitly about normalization, the idea that disabled people's bodies should be physically altered to make them more like non-disabled bodies, as though we are just Platonic shadows, poor imitations of able-bodied perfection.

Importantly, the poem is not about impairment. We do not know from the poem the specific impairment of either the speaker or the person being addressed. It is worth noting that the operation, or series of operations, being described might well be some-thing that the general public would think to be a good thing. Breaking someone's legs to make them straighter, making a disabled person better, doing what the surgeon thinks right. How can those things be wrong? Part of the success of the poem lies in the fact that Brisenden allows no room for such attitudes.

One of the most remarkable and distinctive aspects of the poem is its use of the second person singular. Brisenden speaks as one disabled person addressing another. He also, by implication, addresses a disabled audience, who will share the writer's anger and understand the issues involved. There is no sense in this poem of needing to be validated by the approval of non-disabled people.

As my analysis of Brisenden's poem indicates, disability arts is always to a greater or lesser extent a collective activity. In some cases, such as theatre or dance, it is more or less by definition a collaborative process. Even where artists work individually, for example as writers or as visual artists, they work within the context of a collective movement. Their work is addressed to other disabled people, or performed to disabled audiences.

The growth of the disability arts movement

Disability arts took shape in the early 1980s, at a time when disabled people were starting to organize in cross-disability groups such as the Union of the Physically Impaired Against Segregation (UPIAS), the Liberation Network of People with Disabilities and the British Council of Organisations of Disabled People (BCODP).

The situation became formalized with the founding of the London Disability Arts Forum (LDAF) in 1986. The original impetus for this sprang from a perceived need to set up an umbrella organization to safeguard the financial support for organizations in the London area including Strathcona, Double Exposure, Artsline, Shape and Graeae. At the end of 1985, early discussions took place between representatives of Artsline, Graeae, Shape, Strathcona and Haringey and Greenwich Disablement Associations.

The nature of the organization was changed by Vic Finkelstein, a leading member of UPIAS, and closely involved in the establishment of the BCODP in 1980–81, who argued strongly and persuasively that this new body should not just be a talking shop for a few existing organizations, but should give a voice to the rank and file of disabled people.

At the launch of LDAF, Finkelstein delivered a paper that emphasized the need for both self-identity and collective identity. Finkelstein argued that:

> if we are to make our unique cultural contribution to society then this must come collectively from the people, it cannot be imposed on us by leading disabled individuals from the top down, any more than it could, or can, be imposed on us by occupational therapists, art therapists or any other therapists that are forced on us in the future ... Disability culture ... must develop spontaneously and creatively out of the collective experiences of disabled people. (Finkelstein, 1987: 2–6)

LDAF, an organization controlled by disabled people and employing only disabled people, became a basic model for disability arts organizations. The idea took root that a new kind of organization, disability arts forums, run and staffed entirely by disabled people and creating arts for disabled people, should be the basic model of arts organization for disabled people. As these proliferated, they created a national network of disability arts organizations.

As disability arts developed, it created new ways of delivering artistic work. In particular, disability cabaret, pioneered by LDAF's 'The Workhouse', broke into major new territory by providing a space where disabled audiences could come to enjoy the work of disabled performers. The Workhouse took place at a number of different venues, but there were always two basic ground rules. The event must be fully accessible, or as nearly so as humanly possible; such items as wheelchair access and sign language interpretation could be taken for granted by anyone coming. And there must be a bar.

Paradoxically, this very collective activity, by disabled people for disabled people, created key opportunities for individual performers. The possibility of performing solo as part of a mixed bill rather than as part of a company under a (probably non-disabled) director allowed performers to work up an individual act, and permitted newcomers to gain experience without having to take the weight of a larger production.

It was also immensely liberating for disabled artists to be able to perform to disabled audiences. It enabled them to develop material that was unapologetically disability-based, knowing that it would have resonance for the audience that would be largely or entirely absent from a performance in a mainstream venue.

For a disabled performer, the dynamic of a performance is entirely different when working to a mainstream audience. One has to grapple with prejudice, and sometimes outright hostility, and create acceptance of one's disability before an audience starts to pay attention to one's act. This difficulty is intensified if one wants to perform material that is actually about disability, of which most of the audience will have no experience. When performing stand-up about being epileptic on the mainstream circuit, I personally found a further difficulty: for someone whose impairment is not visually apparent, one has to find a way of announcing it if one wants to perform disability material; audiences, to their credit, are generally unhappy if they feel someone able-bodied is knocking disabled people.

Like the disability movement of the time, the Workhouse brought together people with a wide range of impairments, rejecting the impairment-specific model of organization offered by the disability charities. A typical early Workhouse might have contained blind folk singer Kate Portal, whose act included 'Going Shopping', a song about street experiences with the sighted public, Deaf poet Dorothy Miles, jazz guitarist Timothy Sagosz, a wheelchair user, an appearance by Heart 'n' Soul, the music theatre group of learning-disabled people, and an interview by LDAF worker Sian Vasey with one of the performers or a key figure from Disability Arts, the whole lot MC-ed by me in my guise as epileptic comedian (Sutherland, 1995).

Mental health system users did not play a major part in these early events, though music and poetry performers were appearing at fundraising events for campaigning organizations such as the Campaign Against Psychiatric Oppression and Survivors Speak Out. The creation of Survivors Poetry in 1991 raised their profile, leading to their subsequent involvement in the mainstream of disability arts.

Audiences were equally mixed. This meant that artists who performed work about their own experience of disability would be doing so to a crowd most of whom did not share their specific impairment. This was not a problem. The experience of disability, in the sense of barriers and social attitudes, is a general one, which overrides specific impairment. Thus, when Johnny Crescendo performed his poem 'Where'd you get that leg?', he was writing from the viewpoint of a man who had had polio and walked with a caliper: 'I've known you now for how long is it and/Where'd you get that leg?/Are you alright on the stairs and/Where'd you get that leg? ... ' But the experience of being on the receiving end of intrusive questioning is one that almost all disabled people are familiar with, and the poem was always well received.

It is enlightening to compare this artistic experience with charity advertising, which has also used individual experience of impairment. The charity depiction represents individual experience in order to present disabled people as alone, disempowered, cut off from social contact. In particular, they are *unable to help themselves*. That is the core of almost all disability charity advertising, because its message is: 'They need your help.'

This sort of depiction is generally said to treat disabled people as tragic. That does not strike me as the most appropriate term. The monochrome world of impairment charity depictions of disabled people contains no Othellos, no Hamlets, no Macbeths. We are shown not as tragic, but as pathetic, powerless, unable even to deflect an intrusive gaze. This had been the dominant representation of disabled people for centuries, until we started to take control and depict ourselves, our lives and our circumstances for ourselves. That is one reason why disability arts have been so important: it gave us back our dignity.

With the new opportunities presented by disability cabaret, a number of performers blossomed. The most experienced of these were singer/songwriters who had already been working on the folk club circuit.

One of these was the late Ian Stanton. Stanton was a full-time disability activist, working as information officer for the Greater Manchester Coalition of Disabled People. In performance, he presented a relaxed Northern take on disability radicalism in songs such as 'The Glee Club', which described his experiences as an inmate of a day centre, 'Chip on Your Shoulder' and the classic 'Talking Disabled Anarchist Blues': 'Well I've been called the gentle kind/But no one knows what lurks behind./ Folks don't know that when I'm pissed/I become the disabled anarchist/The wheelchair caped crusader ...'

Another was blues singer Johnny Crescendo (Alan Holdsworth), who, by his own account, had by 1988 been playing in pubs and clubs for twenty years (Holdsworth, 1988). Crescendo's early act included classic blues songs chosen for their disability relevance, such as Ted Hawkins's tender 'Sorry You're Sick' and Big Bill Broonzy's impassioned song about civil rights, 'I Wonder When' ('I wonder when I'll be called a man. Maybe when I'm ninety-three ...').

The opportunity to perform regularly to a disability audience inspired Crescendo to start writing material aimed directly at that audience. What he wrote was strongly political. It included 'Choices and Rights', which was to become a classic anthem of the disability movement: 'I don't want your sorrow, I don't want your fear,/I want choices and rights in our lives./I don't need your guilt trip, I don't want your tears,/I want choices and rights in our lives.'

As the title of that song indicates, Johnny was never one to be afraid of expressing his politics too directly; his work has always been about passion rather than nuance. Nevertheless, he possessed that invaluable ability for a political performer, a strong sense of what it is important to make work about. I have already discussed 'Where'd You Get That Leg?' Another part of Crescendo's early sets was the song 'I'm in Love with my Body.' That is a radical statement for a disabled person to make nowadays. In the 1980s it was quite unheard of.

Disability art and representations of disabled people

One of the key concerns of disability arts in its early years was the way that disabled people were represented, in literature, the visual arts and the mass media. Artists started to create work that challenged existing forms of representation. Women artists, in particular, were influenced by the feminist tradition of making work exploring representations of women and started to make personal work that used images of their own bodies to ask questions about what it means to be a disabled woman. One particularly memorable image from this period was created by the Irish artist Mary Duffy who, as a result of thalidomide, has no arms. Duffy photographed herself in the pose of the Venus de Milo, highlighting the irony that one of the most famous images of feminine beauty in existence is of a woman with no arms, with interesting implications for someone like her.

The type of representation that most concerned disabled people, however, was charity advertising. The large disability charities were widely felt to be damaging to disabled people in two ways. They disempowered disabled people, making decisions that affected their lives without giving them any control in the decision making. And they raised the money to pay for this by advertising campaigns that demeaned disabled people, presenting them as helpless and pathetic.

This inspired a lot of work. Photographer David Hevey drew attention to the construction of charity advertisements, where disabled people are photographed from above, as they look away. They are looked at but do not look back. Their eyes are lowered or their heads turned away, as if in shame at their condition. The mood is heightened by the use of 'dramatic' black and white photography.

Hevey developed a photographic practice designed to counter this. Rather than being possessed by the camera, his subjects were allowed to specify how they wanted to be photographed. Hevey often uses colour and disabled people look out of his pictures, engaging the viewer with a direct gaze.

Hevey took part in the Sense of Self exhibition at Camerawork gallery in July 1988, where a group of photographers took photographs based on listening to how disabled people wanted to have themselves portrayed. Hevey's pictures were portraits of a series of people with epilepsy (his own impairment). He subsequently developed his ideas in the book *The Creatures Time Forgot: photography and disability imagery*, which was accompanied by an exhibition and the set of posters *Liberty, Equality, Disability – Images from a Movement* (Hevey, 1992).

Sculptor Tony Heaton addressed the charity industry itself with his performance piece, *Shaken not Stirred*, exhibited at LDAF's 'Euroday' in 1991. The work consisted of a seven-foot high pyramid of 1,760 charity collecting cans, its ascending ranks of red plastic referring to the hierarchical nature of the charity system. The whole imposing edifice was brought crashing to the ground when the artist, a wheelchair user, demolished it by throwing an artificial leg at it. Heaton commented, 'You get used to seeing people shaking cans, but it doesn't stir us to do anything' (personal communication). Visually impressive, the piece suggested that the hierarchical charity system could be destroyed by the collective power of disabled people.

Disability arts and disability politics

Disability arts was always informed to a greater or lesser extent by disability politics. The involvement was sometimes very direct. Thus, for example, in March 1990, after a number of members of the Campaign for Accessible Transport were arrested after stopping transport in Oxford Street to protest about lack of access to London's buses, a benefit cabaret to raise money for the fines was organized at the Red Rose Club, a popular comedy venue in north London, starring some of the most politically active of disability performers: Wanda Barbara, Mike Higgins, me and Johnny Crescendo (Sutherland, 1995).

Probably the most significant interaction between disability arts and the wider disability movement occurred with the demonstrations against the ITV Telethon, Thames TV's annual rag week, in 1991–92. Telethon had received much criticism for the way it portrayed disabled people as pathetic victims and its implicit message that charity was an appropriate way to respond to disabled people's needs.

Disability artists were closely involved in the Campaign to Stop Patronage, the organization set up to run these demonstrations, and brought a strong sense of theatre to the occasion. Disabled people dressed as beggars, with trays of matches and signs around their necks saying 'Blind' and 'Cripple'. Outside the Thames studios crowds of disabled people milled about, to the accompaniment of speeches from such luminaries as Mike Oliver ('I'd like to say something to the people inside. You do not have our permission') and a non-stop flow of entertainment from Johnny Crescendo, Ian Stanton, Wanda Barbara, me, Mike Higgins (the originator of the 'beggars' idea) and others. In 1992 Tony Heaton's *Shaken not Stirred* was repeated for the press conference announcing that year's demonstration.

The campaign was startlingly effective, in part because careful presswork had briefed journalists well, created photo opportunities and given good quotes. (One of the arts being practised was creative writing.) Much of the media coverage concentrated on the demonstration, and almost all of it mentioned the protest. Telethon, one of the least edifying spectacles on television, had long been protected from criticism by the feeling that it was 'for the Disabled' and it would be bad form to have a go at something that was doing such good work. Once disabled people broke that charitable hegemony – which, thanks to the involvement of artists, they did with great *élan* – others felt free to criticize.

There have long been those within disability arts who felt that it must always be as directly political as this, that only work that embraced the social model of disability was true disability arts. The assumption seemed to be that we should be striving for a kind of disability socialist realism, full of proud, angry and strong cripples throwing off their shackles, with all artists taking instructions from a central presidium, in the form of either the National Disability Arts Forum or the British Council of Organisations of Disabled People.

This extension of the idea that disability arts organizations should be controlled by disabled people was popular with some of the bossier members of our movement, particularly those who were more committed to sitting on committees than producing any creative art.

The truth, however, is that disability arts has always been far more heterogeneous than that. Artists have differing experiences of a wide range of impairments and draw upon their disabilities for their work in a wide range of ways. Any opportunity to see a range of disability arts work, such as an open exhibition, or the annual Disability Film Festival reveals an immense variety of approaches. Even where artists share an impairment and have roughly similar experiences, they may produce entirely different material. Thus, my own response to living with epilepsy has been to write poems describing the experience of this impairment that other people cannot see. David Hevey's has been to take intimate portraits of other people with epilepsy, who can be seen to be a very varied group. Photographer Margaret Mitchell picked up on media images of epilepsy, particularly gratuitous mentions of epilepsy in news coverage of violent crimes, 'in order to illustrate the incredulous and insulting behaviour inherent within media representations when dealing with people who have epilepsy' (Mitchell, 1994: 3), taking pictures where she acts out the images created by the accompanying text.

Though entirely different, none of these sets of work contradicts or undermines the others. They are all part of one picture, three different artists defining different aspects of an experience we all share, with each other and with other people with epilepsy.

Conclusion

More generally, as we share the experience of disability arts, whether as artists or as audience, all of us contribute to a sense of what it means to be disabled, with all the truth and beauty and anger and humour and poetry that goes with that. And we are then able to take that to earlier work and look at it with new understanding. Having become familiar with Hevey's ideas on the direct gaze, it is instructive to look at Frida Kahlo's pictures and see how she looks straight out of every one, fierce and unashamed.

Exactly as Vic Finkelstein demanded in 1987, a disability culture is not being imposed 'by leading disabled individuals from the top down'. It is developing spontaneously and creatively out of the collective experiences of disabled people.

8 The Art of Affirming Identity

Toby Brandon and Alice Elliott

> 'The lunatic, the lover and the poet,
>
> Are of imagination all compact' (William Shakespeare, A Midsummer-Night's Dream, V.i.7–17, 1)

Art is a difficult concept to define. For the purpose of the discussion in this chapter 'art' refers to a kind of conscious use of skill and creative expression that is acquired by experience, the experience of disability being the key theme here. A personal and professional interest in both disability and art on the part of the writers, combined with an analysis of the affirmation model of disability described in detail by Swain and French (2000), provides the foundation for this chapter. It would be impossible in this brief work to explore the diversity of art expressed by all disabled people, for example in paintings, sculptures, drawings, theatre presentations and dance. For ease of presentation, this work will examine illustrative examples that mainly come from poetry and other written formats. It is important to state at this point that the authors do not feel that it is appropriate or necessary to define groups of disabled people by their impairment, as art here is informed by the *lived experience* of disability and discrimination which is shared by all disabled people (Beresford, 2000). However, the authors have taken illustrative examples of work from those people who identify themselves as having a learning difficulty and who are survivors of mental health services. These groups have been chosen in part because of the authors' personal experience where health service use and also being part of a disabled family where one member has a learning difficulty.

Each section of this chapter presents a series of issues surrounding art and disability. We begin by outlining the affirmation model and then lead on to a selective examination of the history of disabled people's artistic expression where poems and songs were used within institutions as a voice of dissent. Next art is considered in terms of its interpretation with reference to therapeutic intervention, purely artistic importance and its affirming role. The collective voice of disabled people through the development of a disability culture is explored and finally the significance of this in challenging the tragedy model and developing a positive identity of disability is discussed.

The affirmation model of disability

The affirmation model is conceived as partly separate from the social model of disability arising from a disability culture of artists rather than academics, its main characteristic being the avid rejection of the tragedy model of disability. The tragedy model (Swain et al., 1993) conceptualizes both disability and impairment within the person as a problem that needs to be fixed, and tends to elicit pity and concern from non-disabled people. Disability subsequently becomes steeped in negativity, which is classically expressed through the media's readiness to refer to people as 'suffering' from disability. This justifies all manner of interventions and treatments in the attempt to alleviate this suffering, provoking notions of repairing or rehabilitating the impaired body to 'normal' or 'whole'. Tragedy here does not only define disabled people in society but becomes part of a 'them' and 'us' culture that also frames what is not disability. In contrast the affirmation model is born from the idea that being disabled has benefits in terms of quality of life, experience and lifestyles. On this subject Swain and French write:

> Non-disabled people can generally accept that a wheelchair-user cannot enter a building because of steps … Non-disabled people are much more threatened and challenged by the notion that a wheelchair-user could be pleased and proud to be the person he or she is. (2000: 570)

At an annual general meeting of a disabled people's organization a woman spoke up stating that her impairment and wheelchair use were the defining characteristics of her life, without which she would not have purpose, a partner, or a profession. This positive identity therefore encompasses both disability and impairment, being concerned with the recognition of oppression. Peters explores this by stating:

> Cheryl Marie Wade, as a disabled woman poet puts it, 'Many of us couldn't fit into mainstream view of the world if we wanted to – and some of us wouldn't want to if we could'. (2000: 584)

This approach goes beyond disabled people purely neutralizing any negative posture to replacing it with a positive reconstruction of identity (Morris, 1991). Disabled people's direct experience is not only valid but pivotal to their sense of worth and self. Affirmation in relation to disability can refer to many different aspects of positive identity including sexuality, group, employment and a heightened understanding of the oppression of others. It also rejects the assumptions of dependency that often shadow disability. Importantly, Swain and French comment that:

> There is an assumption that disabled people want to be 'normal', although this is rarely voiced by disabled people themselves who know that disability is a major part of their identity. (2000: 573)

Art and disability: a history of inspiration and dissent

It is not the intention here to examine in detail the notion that art comes from within the individual's psychological makeup, that is what their creative drives mean in detail to the artist, and what personal factors influence the production of a body of work. Questions arise such as: do people become great artists because of their mental health issues or despite them? do mental and emotional pain necessarily lead to creative expression? and does the artist tap into some place in their deepest psyche providing them with a rich source of expression? If nothing else these questions are prone to lead to an over-romantic, sentimental and potentially patronizing discourse. However, it can be proposed that some of the great painters' work such as that of Van Gogh and Edvard Munch followed closely their contrasting mental health experiences. In addition many great writers such as Blake, Byron, Plath, Woolf, Hemingway, Poe, Tennyson, Keats and Beckett have all at some time been associated with mental health issues. Jamison gives a clear example of this, opening her book exploring mental health and the artistic temperament, *Touched with Fire*, with a poem by Drayton:

> his raptures were,
> All air, and fire, which made his verses clear,
> For that fine madness still he did retain,
> Which rightly should possess a poet's brain. (1993: 1)

Similarly in music, the documented biographies of Beethoven, Billie Holiday, and Kurt Cobain also allude to mental health concerns. However, that said, it is not our intention to retro-speculatively pathologize a selection of great artists. Furthermore, it seems equally frivolous to postulate that art is more worthy or somehow of better quality if produced by disabled people, or even to explore whether different impairments lead to different styles of art. Such outside-in approaches have a tendency to fall into the trap of judging disabled peoples' art, labelling it, explaining its roots, and in doing so diluting its impact and ownership by the disabled people themselves. Taking certain hallucinogenic drugs has been described as enhancing the creative act, by gaining access to an altered state, as explored in the writings of Aldous Huxley (2004). The notion of genius has often been closely related to 'madness'. Edgar Allan Poe writes in his famous story 'Eleanora'

> Men have called me mad, but the question is not yet settled, whether madness is or is not the loftiest intelligence – whether much that is glorious – whether all that is profound – does not spring from disease of thought – from moods of mind exalted at the expense of the general intellect. (1917: first para.)

Breakthroughs in science and philosophy have been on occasion characterized as 'eureka moments' coming from some kind of epiphany, a moment of blending rational and irrational thought (Gregory, 2003). These leaps of belief or faith can be considered as close to moments of deep mental health trauma. The notion that pain might bring depth and meaning to life is a cultural commonplace. Shamans in different cultures have been considered as intermediaries between the natural and spiritual worlds. Halifax writes on the subject:

> Accounts of the shaman's inner journey of turmoil and distress, sung and poeticised, condense personal symbolism through a mythological lens that encompasses the wider experience. Through creative expression, the human condition is elevated, mythologised, and, at last, collectively understood … The withdrawal into solitude through sickness opens the way for the inner initiation to take place. Myth in this case evolves from the ground of the diseased body-mind. (1981: 19)

The history of art is suffused with references to dissent, for example black slaves' singing in the cotton fields being the origins of soul, gospel and jazz. The following excerpt is one slave's perspective (Modern American Poetry website: see References):

> We raise de wheat
> Dey gib us de corn
> We bake de bread
> Dey gib us de cruss
> We sif de meal
> Dey gib us de huss
> We peal de meat

Dey gib us de skin

And dat's de way

Dey takes us in

Brandon (1990) in a chapter entitled 'Songs of Protest' reported the story of Betsy Bell – a woman with learning difficulties who lived between 1959 and 1973 in Brockhall, a long-stay hospital in the north-west of England. Her experience of the hospital was reported as one of physical and mental abuse at the hands both of other people with learning difficulties and of staff. She stated that she was lonely being away from her family and became 'dopey' as a result of the medication she was forced to take. She recounts:

DID YOU EVER HEAR SOME OF THE OLD SONGS WE USED TO SING IN BROCKHALL HOSPITAL?

Come to Brockhall

come to Brockhall

It's a place of misery

Round the corner there's a signpost

saying welcome home to me.

Don't believe it

don't believe it

It's a pack of dirty lies

If it weren't for Dr*

we would be in Paradise.

Build a bonfire

build a bonfire

put the Matron on the top

put the staff in the middle

and burn the bloody lot.

(Sung to the tune of Clementine: 1990: 19)

Both songs bear an ironic witness to an oppressive 'home' environment: one describes the misery of the long-stay hospital and the other the horrors and basic denial of the needs of the slaves. If you impose extreme measures of social control on a group, music and art may be one of the few recourses open to them. Brandon (1981: 20) also produced a selection of writings by survivors of the mental health services, amongst which this poem stands out:

THE BARRIER

He is labelled STAFF

He is sitting there

Or is he really there?

I know he isn't

Because I can see

That he is another person

Just like me

Except he has barriers,

Just one word is written

STAFF

I would be glad

If he removed

His barrier called STAFF

And spoke to me

As he. (Jean Townsend)

Again, this clearly articulates one person's struggle to challenge 'the system' and move beyond professional boundaries and the stilted communication of the medical model. Historians have tended to write out the experiences of disabled people, hiding them from detailed study. Disability art here can provide an indelible record of these 'histories from below'. On this subject Onken and Slaten argue that it is important for disabled people, as they overcome segregation, to hold on to their sense of identity and history of struggle (2000: 110).

Interpreting art

Art for many people is considered a hobby or a pastime; as such, people may describe it as cathartic or therapeutic but not necessarily as therapy. In this sense, art is more a relief from everyday life and an expression of something inside, as opposed to a formalized system of treatment. Art therapy has increasingly been seen as a positive health initiative, being framed within policy as improving outcomes around social inclusion and recovery (Department of Health, 1999). In a small-scale study, Heenan recorded that mental health service users reported that art courses had increased self-esteem and empowerment:

> *Art therapy programmes can significantly affect the quality of individuals' lives*
> *and their ability to recover from mental ill health, yet to date these innovative*

> *schemes are over-subscribed, under-funded and marginal to mainstream mental*
> *health services. (2006: 189)*

Recently art has been increasingly involved in health promotion for various groups via community-based projects. Dooher and Byrt (2003) state, using the classic work on empowerment and education by Freire (1972), that: 'The use of arts in healthcare can also result in critical consciousness raising' (2003: 246).

Art therapy involving many different groups and individuals has gained kudos as the result of a long history of interventions in peoples' lives (Knill, 2004). However, people with learning difficulties have often been placed in therapy groups under the auspices of art: this bastardized form of art therapy in day centres tends to be 'done' on a Tuesday afternoon, ostensibly to help disabled people come to terms with their conditions and situations. Disabled people do not tend to own this process, their time being structured around the art sessions and not the art being structured around their time. The creativity of art, its freedom of expression, is lost and replaced by issues more to do with containment, filling of disabled people's time and 'treating' them. In Arnstein's classic (1969) 'ladder of participation', an overall typology of citizen power, a clear and useful illustration of some of the key issues of user participation within services, is proposed. Provocatively, 'manipulations' and 'therapy' are on the non-participation rungs of the ladder, below tokenism and true citizen power. Arnstein astutely comments that: 'participation without redistribution of power is an empty and frustrating process for the powerless' (1969: 216).

The poet John Clare was born in 1793 the son of a peasant; he spent twenty-eight years in various asylums, dying in one at the age of 71. Patten writes of Clare:

> *For a while he was at High Beech, a private asylum in Epping Forest, run by*
> *Dr Matthew Allen, a physician and writer. Allen was one of the first doctors to*
> *consider treating the insane with sympathy, and he encouraged Clare to continue*
> *writing. In many other asylums such an activity would have been discouraged.*
> *One Peterborough doctor who had been treating Clare for some years decided*
> *that Clare's madness was caused by 'years addicted to Poetic prosings'. (1981,*
> *Foreword)*

This is reminiscent of Rosenhan's (1973) work on 'being sane in insane places'. Members of Rosenhan's research team got themselves admitted to various psychiatric hospitals and were instructed to say they had heard a voice: all were diagnosed as having schizophrenia. Rosenhan describes how the behaviour of these pseudo-patients was interpreted and reframed as continuing evidence of their 'syndrome'. For the covert patients within a psychiatric hospital note taking was described as 'obsessive writing behaviour'. John Clare wrote the classic 'I am' about his experiences:

I am: yet what I am none cares or knows,

My friends forsake me like a memory lost;

I am the self-consumer of my woes,

They rise and vanish in oblivious host,

Like shades in love and death's oblivion lost;

And yet I am, and live with shadows tost

Into the nothingness of scorn and noise,

Into the living sea of waking dreams,

Where there is neither sense of life nor joys,

But the vast shipwreck of my life's esteems;

And e'en the dearest – that I loved the best –

Are strange – nay, rather stranger than the rest.

I long for scenes where man has never trod,

A place where woman never smiled or wept;

There to abide with my Creator, God,

And sleep as I in childhood sweetly slept:

Untroubling and untroubled where I lie,

The grass below – above the vaulted sky. (Clare, 1997: 90)

Clare is part of a history of writers with mental health issues who continued to produce work often in very difficult and oppressive situations.

Art as a collective voice of disabled people

Creative writing is uniquely placed to empower the individual. Through the processes of writing each individual's voice can be articulated and their experiences shared and understood in ways that are accessible. Living through disempowering experiences can take your voice away. Creative writing enables you to reclaim your voice. (Waddington Street Writers Group, 1997: 2)

This group in Durham is not writing here about their mental health issues, but about the importance of the collective process of writing and working together to produce a body of work. The empowerment of hitherto suppressed narratives has become increasingly important; for example the publishing company Parents with Attitudes have produced a number of collections of work on education, inclusion and disabled people (Murray and Penman, 1996 and 2000) which have had a strong impact on the field. They introduce one of their texts as follows:

> We recognise that the stories in this collection reflecting experiences based on disablement do not stand in isolation. They are also part of a bigger collection of stories across the spectrum of equalities issues reflecting a much broader range of experiences of discrimination and oppression within our culture; a collection of stories of difference in relation to power and inequality and the consequences of this. (2000: xiii)

Allen (2005) writes that a major impetus of the disability arts movement is to reject the invisibility imposed on disabled people. It is fair to say that much of the arts movement has focused on the abnormal body and its new power to challenge age-old stereotypes of beauty and perfection, for example the (2006) statue depicting Aliso Lapper in Trafalgar Square. This represents a landmark positive rebranding of disability in the most public of places. Within this context art can be framed as a politically affirming way for the disabled individual and/or group to create a positive identity. Also in terms of mental health Onken and Slaten point out that 'this new thinking promotes recovery and resiliency rather than chronicity and dependency while acknowledging the significant challenges faced by people with psychiatric disorders' (2000: 100).

Tragedy, positive identity and an affirmation culture

In the early 1970s the Mental Patients' Union was formed to fight the 'conspiracy of deafness' that confronted mental health service users. Their quest was to expose psychiatric treatments as punishment, social control and what might be called mind policing. More recently further survivor organizations have formed. In a BBC television programme entitled 'I Love Being Mad' (www.bbc.co.uk/blogs/auch/200604/i-love-being-mad,html) powerful and affirming statements about mental health were expressed, such as 'Schizophrenia is not something I caught, it's something I am.' Another mental health survivor described themself and their collective movement as 'Individual mad miracles who came together to dance, in our own way.'

The Mental Patient's Union campaigned under the provocative banners of 'Kiss it' and 'Hugs not drugs'. The overall message from the group was that they could not engage with society in the way that society wanted them to. The TV programme was full of humour, stressing the commonality of 'madness' and the positive role of art in their lives. Art was framed as allowing them to share a creative reality beyond the reach of the 'sane'. At one point their artwork was displayed in a hospital to directly challenge the medical professionals who treated them. Madness was reported by one survivor as a spiritual crisis. On a 2007 television programme entitled 'The Secret Life of the Manic Depressive', the writer and broadcaster Stephen Fry talked candidly about his own mental health with fellow actors Carrie Fisher and Richard Dreyfus, and British comedians Tony Slattery and Jo Brand. The following discussion illustrates the complex relationship they have with their mental health:

> Fry to Slattery: *Here's a button and if I were to press that button you would take away every aspect of bipolarity which has not caused you the greatest happiness over the years but maybe it's had something to do with who you are, so do you want to press the button?*
>
> Slattery: *No I'll keep it, at the moment; because I am in an equitable state I choose not to press the button but I would like to have the option.*
>
> Fry: *Do you know almost everyone I have spoken to said that. It says something about manic depression that despite it being the greatest killer of all psychiatric illnesses many of those suffering from it if given a chance don't want to get rid of it, and if I am honest I don't. (Fry, 2006)*

In the same vein the renowned anti-psychiatrist R. D. Laing (1967) controversially suggested that madness might be considered a 'breakthrough' rather than a 'breakdown'. For Laing, the mental health issues experienced by people could be considered within the context of a process of personal growth comparable to a kind of shamanic journey. He did not dismiss totally the value of psychiatric treatment but challenged the biological foundations of mental distress and subsequent medical intervention regimes. He saw mental health distress as a process of growth that could herald deep realizations, important insights, the development of wisdom and a stronger identity.

People with learning difficulties have lobbied for change through strings of local organizations. For example, People First states that it puts this into action by the removal of negative labelling and the support of risk taking and rights for people with learning difficulties. People First is affiliated to a number of collective arts groups. One such group is Heart'n Soul based in London, which describes itself as a group of artists with learning disabilities, intent on 'quality, integrity and diversity' (Heart'n Soul' website, 2006). Anjali is a professional dance company, within which all the dancers have a learning difficulty, and its website (2006) states that its aim is 'to show that disability is no barrier to creativity'.

The Lawnmowers is a theatre group of people with learning disabilities based in Gateshead. According to its publicity, 'They research, devise and perform shows that reflect their own concerns'. Their latest DVD production 'combines their own brand of humour with great performances, songs and movement as they move through their responses to the Government White Paper, Valuing People' (Lawnmowers, 2006). Having seen the Lawnmowers perform, we know that their work is full of pride and integrity, attempting to educate with humour by, on occasions, subverting existing stereotypes of disability. It is important to note that although People First is run by people with learning difficulties, not all drama companies and other artistic groups are. They may have disabled actors and dancers but not disabled writers, producers and managers. This is significant when considering who this art truly represents and who controls its final delivery.

The socially constructed assumption that being impaired is a tragedy can be challenged using art, but not by showing that 'despite' impairment or disability art can be produced, for example in headlines like 'Against all odds plucky blind girl wins music prize'. Art can be a medium for exploding these falsehoods. Casling (1994) objects to the idea that there is an art that is intent on the political and an art that is personal: he suggests that the difference is unnecessary as all art is ostensibly political in nature, and in feminist terms the personal is the political. In disability culture the political discourse is of the 'other' but also the 'us', or as Neath and Schriner describe it:

> a kinship based on identification of shared understandings of common life experiences ...(disability culture) ...enables a sense of connectedness that can break down the feelings of isolation and alienation that stem from the belief that disability is a personal tragedy which necessarily excludes the disabled persons from full social participation ... it provides a space within which positive identities can be constructed. (2003: 676)

Culture brings meaning to a society; it is however a nebulous term and involves elements connected to ambience, the ways of doing things, levels of energy, individual freedom, the kinds of personalities involved, values, norms and ideologies (Handy, 1999; Brandon, 2005). The development of disability culture was a direct reaction to the traditional tragedy culture with its negative stereotypes, stigma and pathology of disabled people. Disability culture has been expressed through workshops, conferences, art shows and poetry readings (Barnes et al., 1999). Marxist theorists base disability culture within the valuing and exchange of limited resources and coercion in perpetuation of a capitalist society. Recently theorists have tended to move away from some of these roots (Charlton, 1998) to perspectives based in more feminist and postmodern positions (Corker and Shakespeare, 2002), the latter celebrating the 'politics of signification' where artistic expression can be revolutionary. However, questions still persist. Barnes et al. ask:

> are disabled people able to develop values and representations which are selfsupporting and promote an acceptance of the validity of life with impairment? (1999: 203)

The disability arts movement perhaps offers one such vehicle for self-affirmation. Barnes et al. suggest that:

> the main contemporary arena where a positive cultural conception of disability is fostered is disability arts. While this grows out of shared socialization, it goes beyond the experience of negative social institutions to develop a distinctly political notion of culture. (1999: 205)

Disability art is solidarity in a shared vision of the political importance of art in creating and challenging oppression. It sets up in opposition to the concept of the 'flawed artist'. This is affirmation in terms of the disabled person's individual identity or the disabled art group's collective identity. Hevey writes that: 'The disability arts movement is the first sign of a post-tragedy disability culture' (1992: 119).

Conclusion

David Brandon was a mental health service user and professor of social work. He used his direct experience of mental health services in his work to connect with people and used poetry to express the feelings of despair which both haunted and drove him. The following poem is typical of his critical approach to social work, a profession he loved, defended and deconstructed.

Social Workers

We make a sort of bewildered
anxiety riddled living,
part of a strange fantasy
based on expiation and restitution
trying to assuage some deep
and collective guilt –
skilfully communicating to abandoned children;
homeless people freezing on the streets;
those who've spent most of a lifetime
in psychiatric hells;
old people, mostly terrified,
waiting for their sad end,
at best in centrally heated ghettos;
single depressed Mums struggling

to bring up kids

with snotty noses

on no money –

that they're cared about

by distant bureaucrats and politicians

in black Mercedes

and it isn't even remotely true

as well they know. (Brandon, 1994: 1)

He also used other disabled peoples' writing to bear witness to their struggle:

The staff are few and they are rushed

and mostly they are kind,

they walk me, bathe me, feed my frame

but do not feed my mind. (Poem, written by an elderly patient, found in his locker after his death, in Brandon, 1981: 19)

This chapter has explored the conceptual relationship between art and disability using the affirmation model as a reference point. In doing so it has perhaps posed more questions than can be answered. Hevey (1992) asks whether disability art represents impairment or disability or their interrelationship. Other questions have arisen; such as to whom does the disabled artist present their body of work – their oppressors, the general public or other disabled people? When artwork is produced does its 'worth' depend on whether the artist is disabled? Finally, is it farcical to consider art soley in relation to impairment without considering other social factors such as class, ethnicity and gender?

Art is concerned with the construction and reconstruction of meaning. This chapter has shown that art has been used to 'treat', 'therapize' and 'contain' disabled people. In contrast the meaning for affirmation in disability art is the transformation through struggle and the subsequent development of a shared disability identity. Some disabled artists have used art to take pride in both their impairments and their disability. The expression of art also takes the form of defiance against an oppressive system or a means to educate and inspire others. The paper, the song and the clay allow the anger and injustice experienced by disabled people to be witnessed. This may be generated by their external situation, such as institutionalization or their internal situation, such as a spiritual realization. Art therefore clearly becomes affirmation, acting as an antidote to the tragedy and medical models that are still so pervasive in our society. Art can be used by the artist, audience, promoter, government and the media to affirm, deny and even attack. Whether the artist's body of work stands alone from the artist is a point of debate. This is one of the freedoms that art allows: the artist isn't necessarily the art. The affirmation model in disability art has also been used to express commonality of experience and a sense of shared culture for disabled people. Finkelstein and Morrison write on the role of art within the disability culture:

> *Introducing disabled people to the social role of artistic creativity and opening a debate about disability culture is a dynamic way of assisting disabled people to challenge their assumed dependency and place in mainstream society. (1993: 127)*

A song or a painting communicates through the power of symbolism, identity and empathy. We may value art and therefore we value the artist in our society, so art allows and encourages disabled people to own and express affirming identities, roles and lives. It is important to stress that any art, including whether politically or personally driven, needs to be critically reflected upon. Without this the affirmation model could become an excuse for the production of mediocre art, where everything is valid and beyond criticism. It is debatable whether the affirmation model is distinctly different from the social model of disability. What is suggested here is that the affirmation model is the natural extension of the social model, in a sense the antithesis of the tragedy model.

The cultural identity of disability is born from the resonance of individual experiences of disabled people becoming politicized. Disability art can politicise identity, illuminating and challenging discrimination and stigma. Art historically has been the sanctuary of radical thinkers, dissidents and creative minds. It has always been a fertile ground for the expression of marginalized groups and therefore within any disability organization and movement art needs to be recognized as a way into new ideas and directions. The artist may touch upon issues of identity in a far more accessible way for the general public than the work of many academics.

9 An Exploration of Quality of Life of Adults with Haemophilia

Karen Beeton

There has been little discussion in the disability literature regarding the life experiences of individuals with haemophilia. There has, however, been an intense focus on examining the impact of this condition on quality of life (QoL) within the medical profession. The medical interest in the evaluation of QoL is in part due to the considerable costs of the treatment of haemophilia and the need to justify these costs to commissioners and purchasers. As a result, there has been a growing body of research located within the quantitative paradigm and grounded in the medical model that has examined the impact of haemophilia on QoL. There has, however, been a paucity of research located in the qualitative paradigm. Evidence suggests that the findings of interview-based studies may produce different outcomes to the more medically based standardized measures (Cella and Tulsky, 1990; Sidell, 1993). This chapter will discuss some of the findings of a qualitative study that explored partici-pants' perceptions of the impact of haemophilia on QoL. The chapter will begin by outlining the condition haemophilia, the impairments that may result and the impact it is reported to have on the measurement of QoL. Some of the findings from the qualitative study will then be presented in order to illustrate how having haemophilia can shape an individual's life in a positive and affirming way.

A brief overview of haemophilia

Haemophilia is a bleeding disorder that occurs in males and is usually inherited through an X-linked recessive chromosome but can also occur in individuals with no family history (Rizza, 1997). The deficiency of one of the clotting factors (Factor VIII or IX) can cause bleeds that occur predominantly into the musculoskeletal system particularly the knees, ankles and elbow joints. Severely affected individuals may bleed spontaneously or in response to only minor trauma. The presence of blood in the joint can damage the joint surfaces. This can lead to arthropathy, which often occurs at a young age and may be associated with pain, deformity and contractures. The treatment of musculoskeletal bleeds, in conjunction with a graded exercise programme, is to replace the missing factor by intravenous injection so that normal clotting can occur. In addition, prophylactic treatment programmes are now commonly utilized to increase the circulating level of factor in the blood in order to reduce the frequency and severity of bleeds. Whilst factor replacement has undoubtedly improved the lives of those who have the condition, the use of contaminated blood products in the past caused many individuals to develop the Human Immunodeficiency Virus (HIV) and hepatitis. Although these problems no longer occur, many individuals are living with these co-morbidities as well as other health problems. Haemophilia is therefore perceived to affect QoL due to the physical and psychosocial effects that the condition can impose on an individual.

QoL research in this field has predominantly been quantitative in design, using standardized generic questionnaires which include a range of domains purported to assess an individual's QoL. More recently, haemophilia-specific QoL questionnaires have been developed, although these have tended to be focused on assessing the QoL of children (Bullinger et al., 2002; Manco-Johnson et al., 2004; Young et al., 2004). Overall the findings of the studies in adults have demonstrated that QoL was lower in individuals with haemophilia compared to non-disabled people (Miners et al., 1999; Aznar et al., 2000; Mohlo et al., 2000; Solovieva, 2001; Trippoli et al., 2001; Gringeri et al., 2003; Wang et al., 2004). However, closer inspection of the results of the various QoL domains revealed conflicting findings. In some studies being HIV positive or having more frequent bleeds reduced scores on the measured domains but in other studies these variables appeared to have no influence (Djulbegovic et al., 1996; Miners et al., 1999; Mohlo et al., 2000; Trippoli et al., 2001). It has been suggested that either the tools were not sensitive enough to detect the changes, or it may depend on when the tool was administered or that these issues do not affect QoL (Hays and Shapiro, 1992; Miners et al., 1999; Royal et al., 2002). The mental health domain of the QoL measurement tool was rarely affected. Thus, in spite of physical challenges and possible negative psychosocial effects of living in a disablist society, individuals with haemophilia were not depressed, anxious or unhappy.

At a symposium reported in the journal *Haemophilia*, the question and answer session following the presentations was reported. Fischer et al. (2003) acknowledged that measuring health-related QoL was problematic as it was difficult to separate QoL from coping. Fischer et al. (2003) recognized that the measurement of QoL could be confounded by how well a person had adapted to their condition. She continued, 'you can be perfectly happy being blind and say you have excellent QoL. We would say, being blind was not so good as being able to see' (Fischer et al., 2003: 82). This is a medical perspective that emphasizes the commonly held view that optimum health and an absence of impairments are essential in order to experience good QoL. It also implies that having impairments is a tragedy. This perception lies in direct conflict to the affirmative model of disability (Swain and French, 2000). It also highlights the assertion that health professionals tend to rate the health and QoL of individuals with health conditions and impairments more negatively than the individuals themselves.

From the initial development of disease-specific questionnaires to investigate the impact of haemophilia upon QoL in children, one of the most notable features has been the rejection, by children themselves, of the emotional impact words 'problems with self-esteem, social acceptance or emotional wellbeing' and 'being angry, sad or in a bad mood' as a result of haemophilia. These words were not considered relevant to their condition by the participants although medical experts had identified these emotions as being affected by haemophilia (Bullinger et al., 2002; Young et al., 2004).

It would appear that another approach is needed in the evaluation of QoL in individuals with haemophilia. It was envisaged that a qualitative approach would offer an alternative perspective to the existing body of research and provide a deeper understanding of this complex area.

The study process

Severely affected individuals with haemophilia over the age of 16 years were invited to participate in the study. Participants were offered a choice of attending either a focus group or an individual interview if they did not wish to participate in a group discussion. Focus groups were offered, as it was perceived that they can enhance the richness of the data through the shared interactions of participants (Morgan, 1997). Nineteen participants took part in one of two focus groups or an individual interview. Their ages ranged from 27 to 73 years. Six participants were HIV positive and all carried the Hepatitis C virus. The participants all reported arthropathy in one or more joints and two participants used a wheelchair, due to severe arthropathy. The interviews and focus groups were audio-taped and subsequently transcribed. The transcripts were analyzed using a 'code and retrieve' method (Richards and Richards, 1998) within NVivo, a software program. The data were then interpreted, edited and refined and presented as themes. Drawing on the themes, the following sections will illustrate the positive and life-affirming ways that these individuals managed their condition.

Constructing life positively around haemophilia

Early experiences of haemophilia

People who develop chronic illness in later life are often reported to experience a bio-graphical disruption at the time of the initial diagnosis (Bury, 1982) where their pro-jected life history can be deeply affected by the onset of an illness or chronic health condition and their entire identity as a person is challenged. Yet the findings from the participants in this study support the evidence that many individuals with inherited conditions do not experience this phenomenon (Williams, 2000). Indeed the lives of these individuals seem to be constructed around the condition and may be integral to it. For these participants, finding out that they had haemophilia was not associated with feelings of loss or grief in the same way that a health condition that occurs in later life might be (Swain and French, 2000; Williams, 2000; Reynolds, 2004). The awareness of having haemophilia emerged gradually in childhood:

> I suppose I was about 7 or 8 before I knew that other people didn't get this. My parents never made an issue of it. I was 11 before I heard the word haemophilia and that was only because I heard the matron at school telling somebody. I knew by then I had problems which other people didn't appear to have. (David)

It was also reported that some participants had been given negative predictions by health care professionals regarding future mobility or limited life span. This made them feel quite proud that they had defied medical opinion by still being alive and mobile decades after it had been predicted:

> I suppose I am a bit smug, a bit pleased with myself. My parents were told I stood very little chance of living beyond 7... Later on when I was at school it was reported back to me that a teacher said 'Aren't you going to do something about David?' and another teacher said 'No there is no point, he will be dead by the time he is 19!' (David)

The participants in this study had experienced many difficulties in their early life as factor replacement was not so widely available when they were children, and they compared those experiences with their life now. They recalled the severe pain and immobility associated with uncontrolled bleeds, the limited opportunities to develop social networks due to having to spend prolonged periods in bed or resting as a result of bleeds and the uncertainty about whether they would be able to undertake planned events. These early experiences mirror published reports of haemophilia management in the 1960s–80s (Agle, 1964; Salk et al., 1972; Markova and Forbes, 1984; Hernandez et al., 1989). These experiences could impact on how an individual perceives their QoL in comparison to those early years and certainly seemed to shape how these individuals managed their condition in later life.

The effect of factor replacement

Many of the participants recognized the enormous benefits that effective factor replacement regimes had made to their lives.

> Impossible to describe how living with severe haemophilia with no treatment affects you. That does make a difference. The uncertainty. The total disruption to your life. Increasing disability. With treatment that goes. It revolutionises your life. Like patients on dialysis having a kidney transplant. (Jim)

This was in spite of the problems that had occurred due to the use of contaminated blood products. Even though they were aware of the risks, the value of factor replacement often outweighed any potential complications. As one participant said:

> When they first warned me that I could get HIV I said well look … I have had 20 years of a good life, I would rather have had those 20 years than gone through the hell of not having had Factor IX. So it is trade-off and I am in plus territory as far as I am concerned. (David)

The participants were also well aware of the costs of this treatment and their gratitude therefore caused them to behave in an altruistic manner. This was deemed an important part of 'giving back' to society and to the NHS. They also felt that they had a lot of experience of the condition, that they were in effect 'the experts', and by sharing information and insights into their condition they could improve the experience of others. This was particularly important if they regarded this type of activity as something they were skilled in:

> My main skill area is being a patient and seeing things from both sides of the fence and a certain amount of fund-raising, ideas and working on it with people, policy things. (Roy)

Helping others also helped to maintain and increase self-esteem:

> I will always be involved in something, that's my nature. I wouldn't be here if it wasn't for the NHS or the welfare state. If I can give something back in some way then I should. I would have been dead years ago … It's something I can do, I have a skill there … It also keeps the intellect going, and that's the most important thing as far as I am concerned. An awful lot of me doesn't work but fortunately my brain does. (Des)

Many of the participants also considered themselves 'very lucky' and were indebted to the health services they received. This is in contrast to the experiences of many individuals with chronic health problems who often report experiences of poor and fragmented health services that are not matched to their needs.

Taking care of their joints

In order to minimize the effects of arthropathy, as well as reduce the risks of developing joint bleeds, participants used a number of predominantly problem-focused coping strategies. These included planning, pacing activities and protecting joints. If these conservative measures were unsuccessful then orthopaedic surgery was also an option.

Planning was important in order to enable participants to live the lifestyle that they wished. This could include having factor replacement before an activity to reduce the risk of a bleed. Some participants would plan a 'quiet' day beforehand if there was a particular activity that they wanted to do later in the week. This would help to ensure that they would not be in pain or have to cancel because they had done too much the previous day. Therefore activities had to be more organized and although this reduced the ability to be more spontaneous, it allowed them to do the activities that were important to them. The arthropathy caused some of the participants to walk more slowly than normal so they managed this by setting off for meetings earlier and were more cautious when crossing the road. One participant planned shopping trips so that he did not have to queue and so could avoid standing for long periods. The participants also described how they would plan the most efficient way of undertaking an activity in order to reduce unnecessary walking or strain on the joints. Despite these difficulties, the participants seemed to accept their physical restrictions and adjusted their life to minimize unpleasant symptoms and enable them to do the activities they wished to do. The fast pace of life and environmental barriers of a world designed for the non-disabled person also highlight the need for this strategy.

Pacing activities and taking frequent rest periods was another common strategy to minimize symptoms. This could involve taking rest periods during the day or resting when out walking, which often enabled participants to continue with activities for longer than they would otherwise have been able to do. Others would continue to pursue a particular activity if it was important to them or they enjoyed doing it, even if it temporarily increased their symptoms.

The participants were also very safety aware. They tended to use appropriate equipment and were observant about safety and possible risks in order to prevent problems occurring. As Roy said:

> Maybe I am a little over cautious; when using angle grinders or power tools, I have now gone to wearing a full-face mask rather than goggles. Most people would just wear surgical rubber gloves, I actually wear leather gauntlets. If it does slip I have got that extra protection and it would not hurt so much. (Roy)

Managing and minimizing symptoms was an important part of being in control of their lives, minimizing unpleasant symptoms and increasing participants' ability to undertake activities that were important to them. Over time these strategies were incorporated into the fabric of their life and became normal and routine. Changes in priorities and values may make any limitations imposed by a health condition of less importance to the individuals concerned. Other studies have demonstrated that people with haemophilia have reported that their health was good or excellent despite their impairments (Salk et al., 1972; Rosendaal et al., 1990).

Haemophilia is integral to the self

Participants reported that haemophilia was an integral part of the 'self'. They were not able to imagine how life would have been without it as they had nothing to compare. One participant noted that it was difficult to evaluate QoL because they were not sure if their expectations were the same as those of other people. Planning around various illnesses was regarded as an inconvenience rather than a major compromise and did not prevent enjoyment of life:

> *The problem is that when you have got some kind of chronic condition, you don't know what not having it is like! So when people say, 'How are you?' or, 'Are you feeling tired?' you've no idea what kind of benchmark anybody else is working to. (Des)*

This could also make it difficult to accurately complete standardized questionnaires which often ask an individual to rate perceived difficulty of selected tasks. The participants found it difficult to regard haemophilia as a problem:

> *I can't look on haemophilia as a particular problem really because I am so used to it, I have had it all my life. If it is a problem, who is it a problem for? (Peter)*

Many of the participants considered that the challenges they had experienced in their early life had made them better able to deal with setbacks in later life. Hence they demonstrated resilience in dealing with haemophilia and the difficulties they had to face and this was transferred to other aspects of their lives. This is illustrated by one description:

> *I think it is just my makeup. I think it has been reinforced a bit by having haemophilia and having had to push that much harder to do what I want, you tend to be less likely to give it up. Yes, you can get quite worn out. There have been times when I was a teenager I thought what is the point, but then you move on to the next bit. You meet another lady or some other bit of interest comes up and you think I'll do that and why was I depressed! You just move on. (Clive)*

They were also aware that many of their friends and colleagues were no longer alive due to haemophilia-related illnesses such as HIV, and this had an impact on their view of life.

> I think anybody that has been through haemophilia for quite a long time has to have a fairly hard shell to have survived. That has had an impact. (Des)

They expressed their acceptance of the condition and considered that they had adapted to a life within the limitations of the condition. As one said:

> My attitude to haemophilia has been: 'I didn't ask for it, but I have got it. So let us fight it. It is no good getting upset and blaming the world'. (Jack)

These descriptions demonstrated a positive response to adversity and challenging situations. Participants accepted their condition and focused on what they could achieve rather than being concerned about what was not possible. Disengaging from 'giving up' involves accepting what is not possible and focusing instead on new challenges and goals (Carver and Scheier, 2000).

> I feel I have had a pretty good quality of life in many ways but how I would feel if all those things were taken away, if I couldn't do any of those then that would be a different situation altogether. But so long as I am able to do some things I have a good quality of life. (Adrian)

The participants in this study did not report being angry or depressed as a result of having haemophilia. Some participants acknowledged that they sometimes felt depressed but this was usually as a result of routine life stresses unrelated to haemophilia such as pressure at work or relationship problems. Depression was sometimes an issue for HIV positive individuals. Participants reported periods in their life, for example finding out they were HIV positive, or having to start HIV medication, when they had a low period but this tended to be temporary. They generally re-evaluated the issue or focused on other areas of life.

One important aspect of the adults' experiences of living with haemophilia seemed to be their ability to maintain their sense of 'self' and to maintain their self-esteem and self-identity. In order to do this they used a number of strategies. They focused on finding an area or aspect of life where they could be successful. They often found success in the workplace. They chose friends who had similar interests and aspirations. They focused on their personal qualities and aptitudes, so that they were still able to make a contribution to others and to society. This enabled them to feel valued:

> I found other interests and I found other things to do and I tend to find that during life that things seem to work out in the end. It might sound odd but I am actually quite lucky. I [have interests], obviously I can only do the background stuff like I

will do the computer side, the graphics and the newsletters. You just find some other way where you can contribute to it without having to rely on physical strength. (Clive)

Park et al. (1999) also identified that individuals with haemophilia sought different roles in social activities, enabling them to contribute while avoiding bleeds or aggravation of arthropathy. Often this was a skill that developed as an adult rather than as a child. As children, participants were more aware of being different and unable to participate in activities. However, many participants had used the time that they would have been involved in sporting activities to develop other skills. As they became older, their involvement in sporting activities became less important. The need to focus on other areas of life was then seen as an advantage of having haemophilia:

I found that it [haemophilia] probably was beneficial in some ways, because given that I couldn't participate in sport, I developed my interest in skills like argument and debate, and so I found, well I can't beat someone on the cricket field but I can certainly beat them in the debating chamber, or something like that. (Des)

The findings of this study demonstrated that these participants were able to maintain and enhance their sense of 'self' and hence their self-esteem. Several participants who appeared to have a strong inner drive and ambition in the workplace did not feel that haemophilia had restricted their ambitions. Access to factor replacement reduced the symptoms associated with uncontrolled bleeds and enabled them to plan for the future. Certainly, the memories of their early experiences of haemophilia appeared to have a positive impact on their perceptions of their life now. The participants who were not working had opportunities to pursue hobbies and interests, and to meet others with similar interests. Many seemed to make the most of their lives, taking opportunities to travel, being involved in social activities that did not cause bleeds and aggravate symptoms of arthropathy. Hence they reported being able to lead a full life. One participant, who due to a variety of illnesses was no longer able to travel, did not feel compromised. He now focused on other aspects of life. In many cases the participants felt that they did more and achieved more than many people with no health problems. Indeed having haemophilia seemed to open up new avenues and opportunities that might not have been explored otherwise. As one participant said:

Would I still be doing what I am doing if I didn't have haemophilia? I don't know. I live my life to the full with haemophilia. People with no problems at all lead a lesser life than I do. I think I am very fortunate. (Paul)

One participant felt that his life would have been worse without haemophilia, as it gave him strategies and a way of dealing with difficulties that he would not otherwise have had.

So I can't say it is a bad thing to have, actually! How would my life have turned out without it? It could have been a lot worse because of being without it. (Peter)

As they had experienced more difficult times in the past they felt fortunate that they were not now in the same situation. They could often recall colleagues who had died, whilst they were still alive. These experiences all positively impacted on their perceptions of their QoL.

Implications of the findings for QoL

The findings showed that these adults were able to construct their lives positively around haemophilia, and they therefore viewed their QoL positively. Individuals with haemophilia may, like others with chronic health problems, draw on a range of cognitive and behavioural strategies to manage their condition. These may include constructing their values/expectations around what they can do rather than being concerned about what they cannot do. They focused on areas of life where they could contribute and feel valued. They accepted having haemophilia: it was integral to the self and it was normal for them. Some participants used the downward comparison strategy (Taylor, 1983), where they hypothetically compared themselves with others they perceived experienced more difficulties or were worse off than themselves. They tended to adopt 'selective ignoring' for issues they could not control (Pearlin and Schooler, 1978) and demonstrated mastery (Younger, 1991) by accepting what could not be attained, finding alternatives of value, sharing their expertise with others and celebrating their success in contributing to society through employment or social activities. Enhancement of skills in a particular field, and a refocusing of life goals and activities, can strengthen the individual's sense of self (Menzel et al., 2002).

They also adopted a range of behavioural strategies to minimize the impact of the condition, such as planning, pacing and protection of their joints. The diversity in life and the wealth of opportunities available enabled many individuals to achieve satisfaction with their identity even if they have a less than conventional lifestyle to that which may be perceived as 'normal'. The adults reported that the challenges they faced in dealing with adversity made them stronger and more resilient in managing future difficult situations. They were often altruistic and acted as advocates for others.

These adults demonstrated an affirmative response to haemophilia showing that having a health condition had brought positive benefits to their lives. A number of the participants described themselves as 'lucky' or 'fortunate'. This response was reported for a range of reasons, including not becoming HIV positive, their longevity in spite of being HIV positive, being able to have orthopaedic surgery or benefiting from more effective factor replacement regimes. Certainly research has shown that people who regard themselves as lucky are more optimistic and have positive expectations of their life (Wiseman, 2004). Having haemophilia could sometimes be an advantage, as they reported that they could avoid activities or aspects of life that they did not enjoy.

Conclusion

Research into the effect of haemophilia on QoL has tended to focus on the negative aspects of health, and positive perspectives have often been neglected or not considered valid. The exploration of the participants' subjective experiences located within the qualitative paradigm provided scope for this perspective to be addressed. These findings show that, in contrast to the general view of the medical profession and based on the use of standardized questionnaires that having haemophilia can reduce QoL, these individuals experienced a fulfilling and affirming life. Further research exploring the views of others with haemophilia is needed, to address the imbalance between the quantitative and qualitative paradigms and ensure that the collective voice of individuals with haemophilia takes a more dominant place within research into QoL.

10 Disabled People's Testimonies

Jasvinder, Arlene, Geoff and Alice

There are numerous means, modes, contexts – ways for affirming identity. This chapter presents four testimonies by disabled people. We (the editors) selected this term as it has positive connotations. In the Introduction to a book subtitled 'Testimonies of Resistance', Mitchell explains the use of the term as 'partly due to the nature of the stories, which give examples of struggle against prevailing ideas and practices' (2006: 7). The testimonies in this chapter are examples of struggles of transition towards an identity as a disabled person, against the prevailing presumptions of tragedy. Transition, like testimony, is a nebulous concept of moving from one identity to another – from child to adult to older person, from non-disabled to disabled, from sighted to visually impaired, from one lifestyle to another. Each of the four testimonies covers some biographical details, the barriers to transition, and processes and strategies for coping with, resisting and overcoming the barriers. These are stories of the affirmation of self, identity and quality of life in the face of discrimination, oppression and presumptions of dependency, abnormality and the tragedy image of disabled people that is so often portrayed.

Jasvinder

Bechara samjada nehi – bas damakh firgaiya. Pichley janam deh karm bhughat neh pendah hai.

Poor man, he can't understand – mind has gone crazy. That's our (the family's) karma. It is punishment from the previous life.

This is my mum, Bibbiji, crying out between her wails. Bibbiji had arrived from India when she heard about my stroke and had come to stay with me, in my house, in Bingley, West Yorkshire. She had come to see me, of course, and to give a break to my then wife, Jill, from nursing me, a few weeks after I had come out of hospital. I was almost mute and in a wheelchair, paralysed on my right-hand side, and had facial palsy. Bibbiji was shocked to see me in this state and broke down. I, in turn, started to worry about her ability to care for herself and my wife, as she spoke little English. This led to me suffering my first major epileptic seizure a day after her arrival. I went back to the hospital and my consultant advised the family to leave me alone to convalesce, and guard me from any kind of emotional disturbance. After a few weeks visiting other relatives, Bibbiji went back to India. God knows what she went through, emotionally.

In this testimonial I want to explain how aphasia has led me to address my identity issue, by understanding the implications of being severely limited in using my mother tongue. Aphasia has not just been a disadvantage. In hindsight, the brain haemorrhage and subsequent aphasia forced me to gather the flotsam and jetsam of my life and do some spring cleaning: throwing the rubbish away that I had gathered over the years that was no longer useful and keeping the bits that are precious.

In March 1992, I suffered a brain haemorrhage in the Lake District where I was holidaying with my ex-wife. When I was well enough, I was transferred to the hospital in Bradford, from Newcastle where I had surgery. Although I was told that I would never walk or talk again, I was provided with a (very good) speech therapist to reclaim my English. I had therapy for over two years. In the process I largely lost my Irish accent and acquired a 'Foreign Accent Syndrome', like some people who have aphasia when learning to speak. I had no therapy in Punjabi. I had occasional encounters with other Punjabi friends in Bradford who spoke a different form of the language, Mirpuri Punjabi in Pakistan. My English is now fairly well developed, and is developing, while my Punjabi is woefully inadequate.

'You speak like a white person', my relatives have told me on a number of occasions when my sisters, both of whom had married 'out', i.e. did not have an arranged marriage, were not in earshot. This was not aimed just at my ideas, which are 'foreign' to them, but at the broken, extremely hesitant Punjabi I now speak, with an accent of a Colonel Blimp figure from the British Raj films. Therapy only in English meant my tongue and mouth had difficulty moving in any other way.

Of course the difficulty has not been confined to my own speech, it also affects my understanding of language that others – my mother, other relatives – speak to me. I do not have the stamina to follow conversations. After a few minutes my ears, my mind, are exhausted. Let me say from the outset that my memory in respect to language has been damaged, so words or phrases often are lost unless I write them down or talk to someone soon after the event. If I don't do either of these the feeling, the atmosphere is preserved somehow, and it comes to the surface when something similar happens. I say to myself 'this has happened before' (a kind of reality *déjà vu*), and still cannot remember the event unless prompted but do not remember the words used. What is more, I often have a problem with chronology, the sequence of events as they occurred. This same process is what happens after I have read something or watched a movie. This is true for both languages. But my verbal memory is much better in the second language than it is for my mother tongue.

I've got a complicated family history and this led to an equally complicated relationship with my language and identity. I had for a long time a disjointed view of it. After my stroke I wanted to change my identity for a number of reasons. Until my stroke, I was a successful professional in the field of education. Privately I was known for being funny and quick-witted. In the course of my life, like everyone, I had also done things which I was not proud of. I felt that with aphasia, I had the opportunity to make a clean break with everything in my past, which I did not like, and also give myself a break from the expectations I felt people might have of me: I had lost my linguistic power. I was disabled and epileptic. I was treated differently. I acquired a new role, that of the listener and observer. I felt different. I decided to make a break from the old to the new – a familiar experience for me. I have at least two identities and two first names to match. Up until my stroke, I was known as Binday, by family and friends. Bibbiji named me Balvinder. Binday is a short, informal version of Balvinder. The Sikh rituals for naming were not observed, however. Some days later, my father, Pitaji, feeling uncomfortable about it chose a new name for me: Jasvinder. This is the name on my birth certificate. However, nobody called me Jasvinder. I was still known to everyone, my family, my friends, my colleagues, by the name of Binday. After the stroke, something changed. I wanted to be called by my real official name: Jasvinder. I had a little ceremony and told my friends to call me by my official name. An Irish friend of mine celebrated this in a poem, which I have stuck on my kitchen wall: 'Today is Bin-Day'.

Entering my sister's household in Nottingham was a world apart from my Irish-Punjabi world. I became socialized into a mixed-race, multi-cultural, university-educated household, a world apart from my white working-class council house estate Punjabi/Irish upbringing. I came from a world full of the whirlwind of noise, from an action-packed drama where the daytime resonated with screams and shouts of the adults under stress and the night time was owned by the horrific flik-flak of army helicopter blades above the rooftops. In Nottingham, bookish silence reigned. A provincial boy from a small Irish town, I grew increasingly self-conscious, as I contrasted my sister and her husband's impeccable English with my simple language. In Nottingham, I went to a large comprehensive school. It was so different from the schools I went to in Strabane because it was much bigger. I came into contact with a different type of racism, of a much more threatening kind. The kids at the school couldn't understand my broad Strabane accent, nor could the teachers. I got called a 'Paki-Paddy' and this label stuck. Within a month I had the perfect Nottingham accent. I can't remember having any difficulties with language during those years. I switched easily between all three identities. The problem arose when the separate worlds met. I spoke my 'true' voice, the accent of Strabane, when at home, at my sister's house, and I spoke another vernacular outside at school. When my friends came home, both worlds collided under the watchful eyes of my sister and her husband, or so I imagined. I felt an impostor, living a double life/identity once more, pretending to be English outside of the home, Irish inside of home and Punjabi somewhere else.

Having aphasia, looking inward instead of outward has also simplified my life by forcing me to make a choice between multiple identities acted out through languages. Paradoxically this is an exhilarating experience, and yet also an experience which has a sense of loss, of being shut out of my extended Punjabi family. My maturity has been arrested in it. In fact, this has been a theme of my life. Raised mainly by what, in hindsight, were over-protective women, I have found it easier to let them make sense of my life and let them take the decisions for me. This has antagonized the males in my family who saw me as a mammy's boy. Part of my struggle with my identity is also struggling to grow up. My Punjabi family and my sisters protect me but also keep me around for protection for various reasons, but the Punjabi side of the family do not involve me in any serious discussions – I am too slow – I am not one of the adults. I remain a child for ever. I could have hoped as I matured to resolve the many internal conflicts I had by talking to members of my Punjabi family and getting to know them as adults. Instead I am finding it difficult. It is not so much the younger generation. I can speak to them in English. It is the older generation, which represents my origins and my ancestry. I, like an adolescent, think 'they don't understand my world'. It has always been problematic for me to grow up in the Punjabi world. Now, with aphasia, it seems the choice is no longer mine. I have been refused an opportunity to grow up in my family but have been given a new opportunity to focus all my energies on growing up in my second language.

After my stroke and subsequent aphasia, I developed an identity that is much more independent of my family. A year and a half after the stroke, my wife and I separated. Disabled people from Sikh families from Punjab are well looked after in terms of security and nurture, but for me it is too claustrophobic, limiting choice and challenge. So I chose to be independent and moved to inner city Bradford, where it would be easier to access services I needed. I am happier with my identity than I have been for a long time. I have since moved to Sheffield and made new friends through my interest in justice and I joined the Palestinians Solidarity Campaign. I suppose like the Palestinians who are refugees in their own country, with aphasia I was a refugee in my own language.

I am learning many things through my aphasia and appreciate the insights it gives me. For example, with aphasia I get a sense of an idea and it remains opaque, like seeing through a frosted glass, without precise definition. Or a concept wrapped in cellophane seen from afar. There is so much effort involved in finding the word that often I will forget why I was looking for it in the first place. I then use logic to retrace the steps that led me to the word. I also began to see the value of momentary silence when two people are relating through talking. You need language to define things, to fix things. But the obverse is also true. One cannot take another meaning because the meaning is fixed. The use of language both gives rise to and kills meaning. Words label. Words can name and create meaning, bringing experience and understanding. However, they capture precisely what 'is', not an adage as experienced by that individual at that particular time. They are abstract maps and not sensory reality – moving instantly to objectify without allowing the subjective (i.e. the emotional truth experienced by that individual) to settle. Whereas aphasia allows me time to just 'be'.

Since 1999, I have been training to become a psychotherapist. As such, I am taught to go beyond empathy and pick up emotions, which are pre-verbal. I wonder whether aphasia gives me an advantage here. I have discovered that my energies are directed more towards the emotional than the cognitive, thereby lessening control over what is eventually uttered. In addition, as I find it difficult to speak when emotionally charged, I assume that, in my interactions with people and my clients, I am allowing even more time for speech to form and become grounded. We need to look within and pay close attention to our experience. We can perhaps hesitate to name our experience. Perhaps we do it too quickly, thereby imposing meaning on it and losing a chance to learn from it. I'm no linguist but I think aphasia in both languages helps me here.

Thinking back on what Bibbiji said when she first saw me after my stroke and proclaimed that I was atoning for the sins of past incarnations, I wonder what my family karma is? Perhaps it is about this notion of life as struggle, as punishment. In our family, we are never allowed to relax for a moment, in the knowledge that the next calamity is around the corner. Somehow, I have never seen my aphasia as a punishment. Lately, as I explained, I have seen it as an opportunity to create a new identity for myself, to question the meaning of words; the struggle with my identity is framed now.

I have always been a keen runner throughout my life, running away from stress, often it seemed, towards exhaustion, forgetfulness and finally peace. Aphasia simplified my life, like a run. Aphasia helped me break the family karma. Punishments are not always followed by another punishment – aphasia is not a curse.

(Jasvinder's testimony is adapted from Khosa, 2003. Thanks to Carole Pound for her support.)

Arlene

I was born prematurely and as a consequence of this I developed chronic lung disease. Although my condition first became apparent when I was seven years old I continued to lead a relatively active life until my late teens and early twenties. I ran for our local running club until I was 15. I was never a long-distance athlete but was quite a good sprinter. I was a nurse before my condition got so bad I could not work in this field.

I became a wheelchair user in 1989 after years of struggling to walk and breathe at the same time. At that time I felt liberated by the speed my power chair gave me. When I look back on that initial exhilaration, I now laugh: being a wheelchair user has been far from liberating. I now live within a world where there are physical and attitudinal barriers to my full participation in society.

Life with any impairment is a bit like living life inside a pinball machine. In my game I view myself and others like me as small, round, silver ball bearings, and service providers as immovable objects – as the buffers, which are shaped like marbles.

The plunger is pulled back, and I am sent down the tunnel into the game: around the first corner I have my first contact with this service provider, a large immovable object. I am alarmed; this is an alien world. There are a lot of strange sounds around me, but I'm not heard. The large, immovable, soulless, inflexible marbles have taken over. I'm propelled this way and that, told where to go, when to go.

What happened to my choices? Where is the control in my life? Why can't I be given the information I need to make my individual decisions, to have some say over my own destiny?

I'm on the move anew; it's been decided I need intervention from another service provider. Perhaps, this time they will listen to me. They ask me the same questions. I give them the same answers I have given before. Why? Hasn't there been any communication between the two?

Tick, tock, I hear my life ticking by and yet I have fight to get where I want to go, to have them hear me. Do they hear me? Before I entered the game, I had autonomy, control and freedom. I can see from the wreckage all around myself that others have gone before me. They've been treated in the same way. This time I am conveyed into a safe area; I gather my thoughts and see in the corner of the pen others who have made the journey this far. They are battered, but not squashed.

I notice that they're split into two groups – those like me the ball bearings, and the others, brightly coloured marbles. The marbles are from all different services. These marbles are not the same however, for they don't like the way we've been treated. They want things to change. They have broken free from their own shackles. Their voices have been similarly hushed.

I move tentatively, then with more confidence, towards the marble – this marble is unlike the marble I've previously met in the game, as this marble moves over so I can stand next to it. It does not buffer me away.

Suddenly, something strange happens. More and more like me move towards the marbles and the more movement there is, the more unified we become. Together we are all given strength to get through this game. We share information, we communicate, and by sharing information and working together we urge others, whether they are ball bearings or marbles, to make a positive difference to those they come into contact with.

Marbles must now adapt; if they fail to they must become the debris in the game. No longer is the wreckage that of the ball bearing. The ball bearing remains, shiny and silver, it continues to glow, to flourish, and get to the end of the game in better shape than those that have gone before it.

We begin to move, not as independent entities but as a united force. Together we can prevent others becoming debris in the game. As we make our way onward, our impetus compels others to join us. We are joined by ball bearings like me, who are slightly dented, slightly bruised but certainly not out of the game. They come in all shapes and sizes. We accept all.

By joining together, talking to, listening to, respecting each other, treating each other with dignity, we are a force to be reckoned with. Without integration, those in the game become apathetic, depressed, they're being castrated. With union come self-direction, self-respect, control, autonomy and self-worth.

This game is not simple: hell, life isn't easy, but it's the only life we have. Why should our game be made harder by others who have in the past failed to realize that life is a game of chance? They could so easily become the ball bearing rather than the marble.

Back in the real world, I live each day still having to battle for benefits, adaptations, wheelchairs that meet my needs (not Wheelchair Services' cropped definition of what wheelchairs should do). I have had times when I admit I have not wanted to carry on. Not because my conditions are unbearable to live with, but because I have had poor pain management, did not have equipment provided which afforded me some degree of freedom, or had to wait an intolerable time for key equipment, treatment or services and had no voice.

People with long-term conditions should be shown that their lives may have changed, but life can still have joyous moments, some quality to it. They must never feel that they are out of 'the circle', for a circle without diversity is not a whole, but a sham.

Geoff

I have an eye condition called anaridia which I inherited from my father. I was born with normal eyesight but any knocks or bangs affected it. I didn't know I had an eye problem until my middle teens: I just regarded myself as someone with poorish sight. I went to a normal school and left when I was 14. It was while I was working in my first job as a messenger boy that I began to realize that my sight was getting worse. I was blind in my right eye by then but I could still ride a bike around London. I never worried about going blind, because I expected it. My father, his sister and my older brother and sister all had the same condition. I never bothered to see a specialist; I didn't see the point.

After a while I became an assistant so I didn't need to ride the bike any more. I worked in a big shop in Balham that was OK to start with. I use to cut bacon up on the machine and all that sort of thing right up until I left at 33. But the firm that I worked for, Cullen's, realized that my sight was gradually getting worse so they transferred me to one of their less busy shops. In 1951 when I was 30 I became a registered blind person but I stayed in the shop for a further three years. The only difficulty I had was when someone gave me a list they'd written, but people knew me and they realized I couldn't see. I worked in the shop all through the war. I was called up but they wouldn't have me.

When I was 30 I went along to the London County Council and they said, 'Don't worry, mate, you'll be all right, you can be a Braille shorthand typist.' There was no choice. I wasn't made to leave the shop but I knew that before long I wouldn't be able to manage. A home visitor (which we had in those days) came every Wednesday afternoon on my half-day to teach me Braille. I picked up the system quickly but I was slow to learn to read it.

I had to pass a test for reading Braille and then I went to the West London College of Commerce for a year. I was in a class with six other blind and partially sighted people. I didn't work very hard or take it seriously enough. I used to go out playing cards on a Sunday (though that was getting difficult) and I'd go to the dogs when really I should have stayed at home and studied the Braille shorthand. I bought a typewriter but I didn't practise much with that either. At the end of the course I managed to get a job with the civil service, which couldn't have been more different from working in the shop.

I found it difficult. There was a very exacting typing supervisor there - one of those old spinster types. She used to say, 'I don't know what we're going to do with you.' Everyone was doing about 40 words a minute and I was doing 20 because all the other people had been typing for years. But I managed to get up to 30 or 35 without making too many mistakes. I was much better off financially but I would have preferred to stay in the shop. I'm not a confident person but as long I was the other side of the counter I could talk to the girls and chat with everybody and I felt really confident, happy and friendly. But once I left the counter and went to work in the civil service it was different. I didn't get on so well with people and I didn't talk a lot.

I worked as a Braille shorthand typist in various places until 1968 when the computer programming came along. There was a government scheme to see if blind people could manage. I passed the aptitude test and had six weeks' training. I found the computer programming very interesting and enjoyable It was much better paid too as we were executive officers. I worked as a computer programmer in the civil service for 14 years until I retired. As a result of that I have a much better pension, but socially I would have preferred to work in the shop.

I haven't mixed with other blind people very much in my life but I did join a drama club specifically for blind people when I was younger. I didn't have any social problems there because we were all in the same boat. That's where I met my wife, who is totally blind. We experienced loads of practical problems and it was difficult for me having to do all the seeing – not being able to read print was a real problem. Then Jack, our son, came along and his eyes were OK. He took advantage of us though, which any child would do. If there was something he didn't like for dinner he'd stick it on my plate – he was a crafty devil!

I got my first guide dog in 1964 when I was 53. I wouldn't use a white stick because it singled me out as a blind person. My sight was getting worse all the time but I took it in my stride. You hear people on the television and radio saying how difficult it would be and how awful it would be, but it never bothered me. Socially it was difficult, though. I have a rather flippant nature and behind the counter I used to depend very much on people's reactions. I would make a comment and if they smiled then that would be fine but if not I dropped it. Eye contact with people was very important to me. My attitudes, reactions and feelings towards people, and the way I got on with them, became much more difficult. Nowadays I rarely chat to anyone, because I can't see them. That's the thing I've noticed more than anything else about going blind. I feel out of it.

Alice

I was born hearing but I had meningitis when I was four months old. I was diagnosed deaf when I was about eight months old. My family is all hearing. I am the only deaf person. For about the first five years I didn't know that I was deaf. I noticed that I had a funny box on my chest but I didn't know what it was. But then I noticed in myself I was a little bit different from my sister and my other friends. I enjoyed my childhood. My parents looked after me very well but they hadn't met a deaf person before they had me so they panicked a little bit when they found out I was deaf.

I went to primary and secondary mainstream schools, I saw other deaf people there. There was a deaf unit where teachers of the deaf made sure I got on well with the work and mixed with hearing people. Apart from the deaf Unit, the school wasn't really adapted to deaf people's needs as there were no visual alarms or electronic displays. However, we didn't have a problem with hearing people. I wanted to be like one of them. I learnt sign language in the sign language class they used to provide at lunchtime. I started to learn about the Deaf community, about Deaf identity, because obviously my teacher was a teacher of the deaf. I started to make friends with the other Deaf children, went to Deaf club, after-school club – that kind of thing. I met various Deaf role models who would look after us in the after-school Deaf clubs. I started to learn a lot more about the Deaf community as I grew up. I lived in both worlds – Deaf and hearing. I enjoyed both worlds because I can mix in either world. Luckily I had speech therapy, but it was difficult because I had to repeat words and I got a bit frustrated. I get fed up with it. But I enjoy sign language as well so I can interact with other Deaf people.

My identity seems to have changed over the years. I like to go into both worlds. At the moment I am still kind of half/half. I do believe that I have a Deaf identity because I feel comfortable with it. I have a network there. I have everything.

Deaf people don't like to be labelled as disabled or hearing impaired. It is a term that is used by the hearing world, by hearing professionals. But Deaf people would rather be called Deaf. They believe that they don't need support from the hearing world. They are doing what they can do with other Deaf people's support.

In the Deaf world I always make sure that I am included, but not too much. It could become a problem, conflicts. In the hearing world I do like to be involved because I have hearing friends. Between the two of them I do try my best to interact with both, but not interfere with other Deaf people because of attitudes and political views.

My parents made sure I was prepared for the adult world. They also made sure that I wouldn't panic when I saw what the real world was like when I got older. I did A Levels. I've been travelling a lot. I go out a lot more – from about the age of 16. It was more difficult than I thought, because I didn't have the support of teachers and parents. I wanted to be independent. I tried to overcome all the barriers on my own. So I learnt how to break down the barriers.

Communication was the main barrier. I made sure I could lip-read the person clearly and if there were problems I didn't understand I would ask them to speak clearly and loudly. If there were any problems I'd ask them to write it down or if it was an appointment or meeting I would ask them to provide an interpreter.

I taught close friends and fellow students in classes a little bit of sign language – hello, how are you, how can I help – especially at university. At the beginning they didn't have much Deaf awareness, but they are getting on very well. I'm happy that they have that knowledge of Deaf awareness.

Some people do have a negative attitude towards me. For example, I was shopping with a friend, people were staring at us. But we just ignored it because that is their problem.

I am proud to be Deaf. I don't mind people watching me sign – in the shops or street. But I have had a bad experience with one person who didn't respect my needs. I did ask that person to give me a break, especially an eye break when I am concentrating on sign language all the time, but that person didn't respect me so I asked to discuss the matter. So whenever I have problems with that person I would sort it out. I'd get other professionals involved if that was necessary.

If I couldn't solve it myself I would ask for support. I won't let anyone stop what I want to do.

There are a few things that I would like to do that I couldn't do because I am Deaf. For example, I was told when I was younger that I couldn't be a model. I couldn't do it because I was Deaf. I am pleased I am not a model now. A lot of people thought I couldn't do things like go to university, where I am the only person that is Deaf, and a lot of people are surprised that I do go. But I know that Deaf people can do what they want. They can achieve what they want. Lots of people think that we can't do things, but the only thing we have that is different from everybody else is that we are Deaf.

The advantage of being Deaf is what you can experience – the experience is already there throughout the youth clubs. I've been to hearing clubs and they have loads and loads of hearing people but they don't carry on years later, they lose touch. They get bored and they don't come back to the group because they don't have a close relationship with each other. But the Deaf community is different– it is because we are Deaf and the Deaf community is so small. The disadvantage of being Deaf is that you need to be careful what you say within the Deaf community. Some Deaf people are very strong. They are very assertive, very strong-minded, strong-willed in what they believe and what they want from hearing people. Some Deaf people are very laid back, they accept what they face. They have to be aware what is happening in and around the group.

I have done some voluntary work with Deaf people and I really enjoyed it. My aim was to go to university. I have thought about career goals and that was to improve the Deaf community. I don't mind working with Deaf or hearing people but I have to make sure that my career is on the right path: that I am doing the right things without harming Deaf people.

I want to support the Deaf community and their access to buildings, such as LCD display, to make sure that employees within a place have Deaf awareness, they provide interpreters when needed and provide all the electronic equipment that makes Deaf people more comfortable so that they don't feel conspicuous – because Deaf people don't like to carry things around with them – they like to feel relaxed. I do feel responsible because if I make a mistake it will affect the Deaf community.

I've got a Deaf identity. If I became hearing I'd become lost in which world I fully belonged to. For example, if I became hearing and went into the hearing world that would mean I would lose the Deaf world. I have a strong belief in the future of Deaf people and I align myself with them.

Conclusion

To what extent can these four testimonies be said to reflect an affirmative model of disability and impairment? There is a simple answer: that the whole process of producing a personal testimony is in itself affirmative. These are accounts of a process of making sense of the self and of engagement with the social world, developing understandings through personal transitions in a disabling society.

Three characteristics of the stories stood out for us. First, it is clear that affirmation is not an easily defined single process. Identity is constantly reaffirmed, perhaps particularly during periods of transition. Second, affirmation of personal identity connects with collective identity. It is a process of 'identifying with'. A third recurring theme in the stories is that of challenging, either overtly or indirectly, dominant identities and understandings imposed on disabled people.

Section III

On Equal Terms

On Equal Terms

11

Sally French and John Swain

In the Preface to *On Equal Terms: Working with disabled people*, Sally French stated:

> Disabled people have ... been subject to the hostile and patronizing attitudes of non-disabled people, including health and welfare professionals and those who work for charities. They have been expected to play a particular role of passivity, gratitude, dependency and courage, and have sometimes become inwardly oppressed by internalizing these role expectations. (1994a: ix)

This provides a challenging starting point. It throws down the gauntlet as we turn explicitly to professional policy, practice and provision (the 4 Ps). The overall aim is to address the implications for professionals of a non-tragedy or affirmation model of impairment and disability and set the scene for Section III of the book. In doing so, we build on previous chapters to focus on:

- Presumptions about disabled people and their lives – particularly presumptions under-pinning the tragedy model – suffering, loss, lack and pity;
- The challenges to such presumptions generated by disabled people, either individually or collectively;
- The embedding of the tragedy model within health and social care interventions;
- The alternatives struggled for and provided by disabled people themselves (for instance through Centres for Independent Living);
- The processes of changing the 4Ps towards a non-tragedy view of disabled people and their lives;
- The process of change for disabled individuals and organizations of disabled people.

(Continued)

(Continued)

In the first part of the chapter we briefly review models of impairment and disability as the basis for defining reflecting the problem and on possible solutions. For many disabled people, parents of disabled young people, and supporters of disabled people, supposed solutions are often themselves the problem. As Davis has argued:

> People with disabilities have been isolated, incarcerated, observed, written about, operated on, instructed, implanted, regulated, treated, institutionalised, and controlled to a degree probably unequal to that experienced by any other minority group. (1997: 1)

Thus the first part of the chapter looks back to review professional interventions in disabled people's lives. To complicate the picture further, it is part of the nature, or the politics, of the work of professionals that there tends to be perpetual change. A simple expression of this is in the 'buzz words' that reverberate through discourse around the development of professional intervention, such as empowerment, partnership, person-centred practice, mainstreaming and user involvement. It is to this that we turn in the next section of the chapter. Finally we conclude by turning to the implications for professional intervention, looking from an affirmative non-tragedy orientation.

Understanding disability and impairment

The literature is replete with discussions of different ways of understanding disability and impairment. Priestley (2003) provides a kind of model of models. He recognises four. There are two individual models, biological and psychological, and two social models, structural and cultural. The present book has also concentrated on four models: the individual/medical model; the social model; the tragedy model; and the affirmative/non-tragedy model.

In the context of the present discussion, it is necessary to point out that these models of disability and impairment are just that, and are not models of professional intervention. They are, in essence, models of 'the problem'. There are associated general implications and principles but the models are not blueprints. The medical model remains dominant in professional policy, practice and provision. Given that the model is generated by and for professionals, this is hardly surprising. Also given that the problem is defined and understood in terms of individual impairment, defect and abnormality, the clear implications are in terms of care and cure. Indeed the establishment of a whole range of professions, and the professionalization of western society, is grounded in and justified by this foundation. This was evident in the huge expansion of many professions when the welfare state was founded (Hughes and Lewis, 1996). On the one hand, it is the basis of interventions which many disabled people would acknowledge are essential to their existence and even their quality of life. There are numerous specific examples, including the use of injections of insulin to control blood sugar level for people with diabetes and the use of chemotherapy to cure some forms of cancer.

On the other hand, this basis of intervention has been critiqued on a number of grounds. At the most extreme, it is seen as justifying the elimination of disabled people through the abortion of impaired foetuses. As a midwife recently put it, 'better a dead baby than a disabled baby' (personal communication). It has also been the foundation and justification for treatment that is experienced by disabled people as demeaning, abusive and oppressive. The evidence from research and the writings and recollections of disabled people suggest that client–professional relationships are varied but have often been experienced negatively by disabled people. To an extent, we are looking back at this point, as it is these experiences that provide a foundation for analyzing the more recent developments.

Wendell (1996), for instance, refers to the power of professionals to undermine people's beliefs in the reality of their bodily experiences as 'epistemic invalidation'. Straughair and Fawcitt (1992) report that the young people with arthritis they interviewed were sometimes accused of being neurotic when their symptoms did not fit into neat diagnostic slots. Doubt can be cast on immediate experiences unless they are confirmed by authorized medical descriptions.

Disabled women have reported numerous demeaning experiences. Lonsdale relates many harmful experiences of hospital treatment and medical care. This particularly concerned doctors, who were often perceived by the women as being nothing more than 'groups of anonymous men' (1990: 89). The evidence suggests that many disabled women who are repeatedly subjected to such degrading treatment experience damaged self-esteem. Another common complaint about health and welfare professionals has been their lack of concern with emotional issues. Morris interviewed women with spinal cord injuries. One woman said, 'There is no space allowed for us to express our grief … There is often pressure put on us to "cope" and if we fail to live up to the standard demanded of us we are categorized as a "problem"' (1989: 24).

There are broader critiques of the professional/service system that suggest that problems are ingrained within the system. There are large inequalities in health, with those of the lowest socio-economic status having the worst health. Certain groups in society such as women, old people, people from ethnic minorities and disabled people, are also disadvantaged partly because of their over-representation in the lower socio-economic groups. There are also regional variations in health status (French, 1997). Furthermore, in Britain as in most countries of the western world, these inequalities are increasing (Department of Health, 2001a). Robert and House state that

> Socio-economic inequalities in health have been observed persistently over the course of human history. These differences are manifest across individuals, communities, and societies, and recent analyses suggest that for the most part they have increased over the past century, and even in the past few decades …The nature and size of these inequalities make them arguably the major problem of population and public health. (2000: 115)

Furthermore, the critique of professional intervention based on the experiences of disabled service users, and indeed of some professionals, reaches deep into the professional system. From this viewpoint, services are certainly not rights-led or even needs-led, but resource-led. This puts professionals in the position of gatekeepers, with the allocation of scarce resources as the prime dynamic of intervention. The provision of direct payments, for instance, can be experienced as driven by a resource-led, or administration-led, model. Direct payments, in origin, can be seen as generated by a social model of disability, being initiated and campaigned for by disabled people to increase their control and choice of services. Yet the day-to-day reality is resource-based and in the hands of the very authorities who have a vested interest in retaining their own control and power in regulating choice. Assessment of the individual dominates service provider/service user relations. Professionals are put in the position of what can be characterized as 'time and motion experts'. How long does it take to have a bath, eat a meal, go to the toilet? In the allocation of resources the dominant model is certainly not the social model. A system model predominates, if indeed it can be called a model as such. Davis argues that the system is 'pregnant with career opportunities', for non-disabled professionals, and:

> At this juncture, our lives are still substantially in their hands. They still determine most decisions and their practical outcomes. The Community Care (Direct Payments) Act (1996), again conceded only after years of hard campaigning by the disabled people's movement, offers some of us the bitter-sweet taste of professionally restricted freedom. The control that our professional guardians and gatekeepers hold over our access to it reflects the way in which the decision-making process has been carefully reinforced by ensuring that the climate of ideas that surrounds the making of disability policy is also under their influence. (2004: 204)

Analyzing the relationship between models of disability and impairment and professional intervention, two interrelated lines of critique come to the fore. First, there is no simple divide between understanding 'the problem' and evaluating 'solutions'. For many disabled people the professional services are part of the problem. Second, the relations between service providers and service users are shaped by and formed within a system of power relations that is served by an individual model of disability.

Changing professional policy, practice and provision

The professional literature is replete with notions of changing professional services. Ideas of 'changing practice' and 'new ways of working' feed the view that 'things are getting better' from the standpoint of service providers, managers and policy makers at least. In this section, given the range and scope of the relevant literature, we have taken a particular focus, looking first at three key concepts of change – empowerment, user involvement and partnership – but then concentrating on the barriers to change.

The term 'empowerment' has many meanings and, as Gomm suggests, has become something of a buzz word, used differently in different contexts by different people to promote their own ends. He writes:

> What can we do with a term which on the right of politics can mean privatising public services, and on the far left can mean abolishing private services; which can mean all things to all men, and something different again to some women? (1993: 6)

Defining empowerment, however, Thompson is succinct:

> We can identify its core element as a process of helping people gain greater control over their lives and the sociopolitical and existential challenges they face. (1998: 211)

Whatever the specific definition, the term 'empowerment' is ubiquitous. It pervades academic and professional literature, policy statements emanating from organizations of disabled people, as well as large-scale charity organizations for disabled people and professional organizations.

User involvement has been closely associated with notions of empowerment but has broader political associations. The development of user involvement in services for disabled people arose in Britain in two main ways. Following the election of Margaret Thatcher as Conservative Prime Minister in 1979, there was a shift towards a market ideology in health and social care. A quasi-market was introduced into health and social services to allow some degree of choice for patients and clients, who were now regarded as consumers. The idea was that services would be 'needs-led' rather than 'service-led' and that disabled people and other service users would be assessed for individual 'packages of care' within a 'mixed economy of welfare' including private, voluntary and statutory services (Hughes and Lewis, 1996; Furgusson et al., 2004).

These changes were backed by legislation and various policy documents from the Department of Health, in particular the Children Act (1989) and the NHS and Community Care Act (1990). User consultation and collaboration in service planning and delivery was made mandatory in these Acts. Managers were, for example, required to consult with consumers regarding community care plans. These changes reflected the consumerist ideology of the political right and were viewed as a way of cutting costs, providing more flexible services and reducing state involvement (Beresford and Croft, 2000). In 1997 these policies were, in essence, continued in New Labour's modernization agenda for health and social care (Mercer, 2004; Carr, 2004). As a result of these policy changes the 1990s saw a considerable growth in user involvement initiatives, particularly in the social services, where thousands of disabled people now participate in a range of activities (Carmichael, 2004).

The term 'partnership' can also be used to denote the inclusion of disabled people's voices in decision making in the professional intervention process. This is the principle of working with rather than on people. Thompson lists various features that are needed to form a partnership:

- identifying problems to be tackled, issues to be addressed, goals to be achieved;
- deciding what steps are to be taken and who needs to do what;
- undertaking the necessary work through collaboration and consultation;
- reviewing progress and agreeing any changes that need to be made to the agreed course of action;
- bringing the work to a close if and when necessary;
- evaluating the work done, highlighting strengths, weaknesses and lessons to be learned. (1998: 213)

In recent policy developments, partnership has been a dominant concept signifying the attainment of greater equality in professional–client relations generally. Defining the concept of partnership, however, is difficult because partnership means different things to different groups of people. Broadly, it refers to organizations or individuals working together or acting jointly. Partnerships between professionals and clients are predicated on some expectation of an increase in choice for those receiving services.

Any real choice, however, may be a mirage as choice can be seen as a threat by professionals who act as gatekeepers by continuing to make the decisions about access to provision. Gibbs states:

> Words like 'empower' and 'enable' (even 're-able', which has entered the modernisation programme like a mystery virus) are used in the sense of something that can be prescribed. This usage must be flatly refuted: from the moment that someone presumes to prescribe and manage another's 'empowerment' they prevent it; from the moment they ask 'how can I empower this person?' they begin to do the opposite. (2004: 149)

Many practical, organizational and cultural barriers need to be addressed if empowerment of disabled people, user involvement and partnership with disabled people in health and social care services are to become a reality. A central issue is the unequal power relationship between service users and professionals and managers (French and Swain, 2001; Swain et al., 2004). Carr asserts that 'Power issues underlie the majority of identified difficulties with effective user-led change' (2004: 14) and that 'dissatisfaction and even conflict may be an inevitable part of the user participation process' (2004: 18). Similarly Priestley says that:

> It is impossible to discuss user participation without reference to power. If providers are committed to increasing user power then they must contemplate a corresponding reduction of their own power. (1999: 158)

The power imbalance between disabled people and professionals and managers extends to the meaning of important concepts that affect disabled people's lives. Disabled people and professionals tend, for example, to have a very different idea of the meaning of 'care' and 'independence', with the view of professionals and managers predominating and being translated into policy and practice (French and Swain, 1998; Carr, 2004; Finkelstein, 2004; Goble, 2004).

Beresford et al. (2000) believe that users of services need to be involved in defining the meaning of 'quality', as their definition is fundamentally different from that of service agencies. Priestley states that:

> Definitions of quality (used to judge both disabled people's quality of life and the quality of the services available to them) are derived from and determined by a variety of dominant and oppressive social values about the role of disabled people in society ... the social construction of 'quality' is intrinsically bound up with the social construction of 'disablement'. (1995: 11)

Similarly, Beresford et al. believe that views about quality in services are based upon cultural and professional assumptions that are underpinned by paternalism rather than on the perspectives of those who use the services, which are based on rights. They state:

> It seems likely that service users will want to avoid coming up with any predetermined set of quality standards. Rather they are more likely to see quality as the extent to which services enable individuals to meet their own aspirations, which will vary from person to person, and as the extent to which they enable people to enhance control over their own lives. (1997: 78)

A further way in which inequality of power is apparent in health and social care services is in the setting of agendas. These are usually set by professionals and managers rather than disabled people themselves (Carr, 2004). Furthermore, the involvement of and partnership with disabled people are usually dependent upon resources and adequate funding, for example accessible and affordable transport and physical access to premises.

Many disabled people want to be involved with the services that shape their lives and it is now rare for community care professionals and managers to ignore them entirely in the planning and delivery process (Beresford et al., 2000). There are, however, competing agendas and those of professionals and managers are usually given priority. Whereas service providers are concerned with budgets, policy and the smooth running of organizations, the aim of disabled people is to fundamentally change, not only the services they receive, but society itself. This leads to conflict because, whereas the professional approach starts with 'the system' and how it can be adjusted, the approach of disabled people is concerned with changing the reality of their lives. As Croft and Beresford note:

> Service providers are primarily concerned with meeting the political, economic and managerial requirements of their agencies and services. The concerns of service users are at once more personal and broader: They are committed to improving the quality of their lives, reflecting inappropriate provision which restricts what they can do and seeking appropriate support to live as they want to. (2002: 388)

A non-tragedy approach to services

In challenging the presumptions of tragedy built into and perpetuated by professional intervention, a non-tragedy view addresses power relations at both the personal and the interpersonal levels and the reverberations throughout professional and service systems. To engage with this we shall look towards two recent research projects. The first examined centres for independent living (CILs) and the work of disabled people as service providers (Barnes and Mercer, 2006). The second explored disabled people's advice to professionals in their moves towards 'working in new ways' (French, 2004).

CILs are a particular type of self-help organization, exclusively run and controlled by disabled people themselves. They provide a new and innovative range of services and support systems designed to enable people with impairments to adopt a lifestyle of their own choosing, in contrast to other professionally dominated provision that has focused almost exclusively on medical treatments and therapies within institutional settings. Decision making and working practices in CILs are controlled by disabled people who do not regard disability as an individualized tragedy but as a civil rights issue. Their work is geared towards the fulfilment of disabled people's needs on their own terms and viewing disabled people as active, capable citizens who are restricted, not by impairment, but by a disabling society.

Derbyshire CIL set out and worked towards meeting seven needs, seen as putting the social model into action:

- information
- counselling
- housing
- technical aids
- personal assistance
- transport
- access

Two main themes emerged in the research conducted by Barnes and Mercer (2006): choice and control; and peer support. User-led organizations were seen by participants as far more responsive to their needs both in terms of what was on offer and how it was offered. They felt that they had a greater choice of services and, equally important, more control over how they were delivered. All the participants considered the services to be far more aware of the problems faced by disabled people and, consequently, more responsive to individual need. Furthermore, having the opportunity to meet other disabled people was regarded as of immense benefit by the overwhelming majority.

In relation to a non-tragedy approach the CILs have a number of implications:

- Their work speaks directly to disabled people's choice and control over services and intervention, grounded in user-led organisations.
- They speak too to the non-disabled/disabled social divide. The non-tragedy model is founded in experiences of impairment and disability and the self-empowerment to confront presumptions of tragedy.
- The work of the CILs also gives expression to and translates into action the collective and shared experiences of non-tragedy. The tragedy view is quintessentially individual.

Research by French (2004) also provides food for thought in exploring a non-tragedy approach that has clear implications for developing professional policy, practice and provision. As in considering CILs, changing power relations is predominant. A number of principles emerged.

Be yourself

Sue said:

> Forget you're a therapist – just be yourself. I don't mean forget all your training – but be yourself. Don't be afraid of showing the real you because that's what makes people respond, when they're ill they respond more easily if the therapist is being real. (French, 2004: 103)

Don't presume disabled people desire normality

Kate wants therapists to stop focusing on 'normality':

> What concerns me most of all is this focus on trying to make me 'normal'. I get that from all the therapists. I get a lot of referrals of 'this may help' and 'that may help'. They had a massive case conference before the adaptations – it was a case of 'how normal can we make her first? Are the adaptations necessary?' (French, 2004: 103)

Kevin, looking back on his treatment by speech and language therapists, also feels that striving for 'normality' can be misplaced:

> I do question the years of not enjoying food and getting to a point when I dreaded mealtimes. But now I think, 'This is me. This is what I do. I've made a mess on my shirt and I don't give a toss. It can be cleaned up. Just eat for the pleasure of eating and to hell with the rest'. A by-product of too much therapy and too much intervention is that you go through a period when you're scared of your own shadow, but then you reach a point when you say 'tough'! If I spill my coffee I'm now more interested in the pretty pattern it makes. (French, 2004: 104)

Recognize disabled people's expertise

Sandy states:

> The biggest thing is about asking and not telling. They need to get into the habit of asking what would be helpful. They don't seem to enter into a dialogue – we respect them far more if we can have an equal partnership in the challenge we're both facing. I would expect a person to be trained to the task and have an excellent knowledge base, and I would expect to have an exchange of knowledge – theirs would be knowledge from their training and mine would be about my own body, and my lifestyle. I would expect the therapist to hear me. I would expect them to be creative. (French, 2004: 104)

Recognize the constraints within the system

Sandy empathized with the conditions under which therapists work:

> Creativity is a big thing and sadly because of time constraints and budgetary constraints some therapists have their creativity stifled. The systems don't help therapists to be creative and relaxed. (French, 2004: 104)

Maintain integrity

Kevin urged therapists to keep to their principles:

> When you leave education, when you've got your qualification, be aware that the people you work for will try and make you conform to the traditional way of working. You may need to do that initially, but try not to allow yourself to become corrupted by it. Keep your integrity because when you get a bit higher up the ladder, and get a bit of power, you can try to change things. (French, 2004: 106)

Actively listen to disabled people

Kate puts the point succinctly:

> I want them to say, 'What sorts of things would help you to lead a full life in the context of your impairment?' It's either, 'you're disabled and what can we do to make you better' or 'you're OK'. Nobody says 'What would make a better life?' That's what I would like. (French, 2004: 104)

Relinquish power

Kevin believes that professionals need to relinquish their power and that fundamental changes are needed in therapy education and practice:

> Users should have more power. Until you give users real power, real control, we'll get nowhere ... there's an awful lot of people with a lot of vested interests ...The only way to do it is to get much more input from disabled people into the training. It would be a national scandal if men did a whole load of training on women's issues, it would be unheard of for a group of white people to give equality training on race, but medical people do their training without coming up against it, without being challenged ... Let's get away from the medical model, not only in training, but in practice. Let's get a divorce between the medical profession and therapists. Let's get them out from social services as independent professionals with skills and knowledge ... they're in a hierarchy and the doctors don't want to let go. (French, 2004: 105)

Conclusion

In this chapter we have begun to explore the implications that a non-tragedy/affirmative view of disability and impairment might have for professional policy, practice and provision. A non-tragedy view demands critical reflection on professional intervention, rather than offering a well-established blueprint. For us, it is part of and builds on a social model orientation, with the imperative of changing the power relations between service users and providers towards control by disabled people of the policy, practice and provision that shape their lives.

The establishment of a non-tragedy approach faces considerable institutionalized barriers, including vested interests in maintaining and justifying the predominance of medical/individual/tragedy models; the ingrained non-disabled presumptions about the existence, lives, characteristics, needs and desires of disabled people; and the ethos of the system to maintain, justify, perpetuate and enforce the status quo. Nevertheless, the imperatives and mandates for fundamental change are equally apparent. The following chapters turn to possibilities for a non-tragedy approach in specific professional arenas. Where do the possibilities for control by disabled people in establishing affirmative disabled identities lie?

Some key questions to address in section 3

Activity

This section takes a different, perhaps unique, approach in a disability studies text to examining the issues in professional policy, practice and provision. The authors of these chapters were approached as practitioners, or as involved in service provision in some way. They were each sent a draft copy of the present chapter, and asked to explore the implications for their particular arena. We suggest that, having just read the chapter, you undertake a similar exercise. Select a profession (your own professional area as a practitioner or trainee) or a professional area you have experienced as a service user, and note any thoughts in relation to professional practice working with disabled people. Again this is a good activity to share with a group of colleagues or fellow students.

Questions

The chapters in this section explore the implications of an affirmative model of disability and impairment for professional policy, practice and provision. As you read spend some time thinking about, and if possible discussing, your reactions to this. You might find it helpful to consider the following.

1   One view put forward by professionals is that things are changing in their work with disabled people, often for the better but sometimes worsening. List what you consider to be the main changes in policy in recent years.

2   A concern for many professionals, and indeed service users, is what are seen as gaps between policy and actual practice. List what you see as examples of such gaps in your particular area.

3   As you may already have noted, health and social care buzzes with concepts of change (sometimes referred to as buzz words). Notions of empowerment and partnership are omnipresent examples. What meaning do these concepts of professional practice have for disabled service users? What direct evidence do you have, or can you find, of their views?

4   This book is multi-professional on the straightforward basis that a number of professionals have contributed as authors of chapters in this section. Notions of multi-professional practice (and related concepts such as 'joined up practice'), however, are particularly prevalent in health and social care and go well beyond a simple question of the numbers of different professions involved in the provision of services for disabled people. Indeed, it could be argued that the very number of professions involved is in itself a barrier to developing multi-professional practice. Though the authors of the chapters in this section were not specifically asked to address issues under this umbrella, make a note of any discussion points and examples given that are relevant to multi-professional practice. You might draw your own conclusions from the notes you make. What are the implications of the affirmative model for multi-professional practice? Looking from the viewpoint of disabled service users, what are the possible benefits and difficulties resulting from multi-professional practice?

5   In professional practice disability issues can be encompassed within a broader remit such as 'equality and diversity'. There are numerous questions that can be asked in this context. First, what organisational structures have been put in place in the context in which you work or have experience? What strategies have been put in place to address issues of 'equality and diversity', such as disability or race equality training? And, in the context of this book, what are the consequences of equality and diversity for disabled service users?

6   Finally, building on the social model, the affirmative model of disability inherently challenges the power that professionals have over disabled people's understanding of themselves, their lifestyles and quality of life. As you read the chapters in this section critically reflect on your personal position as a professional, or trainee, or indeed service user, as a provider of services for disabled people.

12 In Practice from the Viewpoint of an Occupational Therapist

Elaine Ballantyne and Andrew Muir

> *Occupational Therapy enables people to achieve health, well being and life satisfaction through participation in occupation … The British Association of Occupational Therapists (BAOT) is the professional body and trade union for 24,000 occupational therapy personnel in the UK. The College of Occupational Therapists (COT) … is a wholly owned subsidiary of the BAOT. It is primarily involved with the setting of professional and educational standards, as well as the promotion of research, evidence-based practice and continuing professional development. COT (2002: 2)*

Occupational therapists are beginning to appreciate that a range of new questions has emerged concerning the way in which they practise. These have emerged as a result of changes in social policy, disability studies and challenges to dominant discourses generated by disabled people and their organizations. There is some evidence in the professional literature that occupational therapists are beginning to reflect on how to respond to disability studies' developing critique. Craddock acknowledged that 'further work is now required to ensure that occupational therapists' response to the perspective of the disability movement is both adaptive and affirmative' (1996: 77). Kielhofner identifies a number of questions 'raised by disability studies that will need to be addressed in practice, education and research' (2005: 487).

This chapter will identify some of the key questions emerging for occupational therapy policy, provision and practice from a consideration of the implications of the affirmative model described by Swain and French (2000).

Implications for professional policy

Developments in disability theory (Campbell and Oliver, 1996; Oliver, 1996; Wendell, 1997; Swain and French, 2000) are key drivers in the need for occupational therapy to reconceptualize itself (Pollard et al., 2005). There is an evident need for occupational therapy to develop an effective response at a policy level to the profound challenges posed to the way in which it constructs its ideas of disability and impairment. It is not intended to suggest specific responses to the affirmative model of disability. Rather, it is proposed that the occupational therapy profession use the emergence of the affirmative model as an opportunity to engage proactively with disability theorists, disabled people and their organizations in a process of discussion, debate and reflection. This approach would give real substance to occupational therapy's key tenet of working in partnership with people, but would be undertaken at a policy rather than an individual level. It would also represent an effective response to the legitimate challenge of disabled people – 'nothing about us, without us' (Charlton, 1998). Pollard et al. propose that, 'by forming alliances with marginalized groups, occupational therapists can develop practice … which accommodates their values and beliefs. Occupational therapists can use theories and tools for change without unquestioningly engaging the biomedical framework for health and social care' (2005: 525).

From an organizational perspective a parallel can be drawn between the occupational therapy profession and Handy's frog. Handy (1990), a management theorist, uses a frog in a tin of water as a metaphor to illustrate how some organizations are unable to adapt to changes in the external environment. The frog's physiology makes it unable to recognize that the water temperature is increasing and it eventually boils. The absence of a coherent response on the policy level increases the likelihood that, as Abberley suggests, OT, despite what may be the best intentions on the part of its practitioners, serves to perpetuate the process of disablement of impaired people (1995: 222).

From a sociological perspective, policy can be seen as the external manifestation of a profession's ways of knowing. All professions are involved in the production of knowledge that can structure modes of thinking and influence everyday consciousness (Mills, 1956). As a consequence of their powerful position in society, professions' ways of knowing are so deeply embedded in people's consciousness that the cognitive frameworks used to understand issues are seen as self-evident and rational. The following example may help illustrate this idea.

Read the following information on a person and then reflect on what you are thinking and feeling.

John is doubly incontinent. He is vocal but non-verbal, that is he can make noises but cannot communicate through normal speech. He is almost totally dependent upon his carer for all his daily living needs. John finds it very difficult to eat a meal or to walk without some form of assistance. He has poor hand/eye coordination and a limited ability to grasp objects.

- Did you assume that John was a disabled person? Why?
- Would your view change if you were told that John was, in fact, 18 months old?
- Does the example reflect the way in which disabled people are typically described as a series of deficits?
- Why is being unable to eat a meal without assistance seen as being 'normal' or value neutral for a person 18 months old and seen as a disability in a person 18 years old?
- Where do your ideas of 'normality' come from? Are they self-generated? Are they the result of a complex and unconscious process of socialization? Which groups in society have the power to define 'normal'? Is this knowledge neutral? Does it serve the interests of powerful groups within society?
- Does this knowledge become accepted as a commonsense way of understanding the world?

Esland suggests that 'many of the dominant categories of thought which permeate our commonsense attitudes – as well as the power to enforce them – are to some extent traceable back to the political organisation of particular occupations' (1980: 216) and that it is accepted that professions can legitimately produce knowledge for society as a whole.

The development of professional policy reflecting the affirmation model could potentially contribute to new 'ways of knowing' impairment and disability within wider society. Instead of 'embodying the ideology of the "few" who hold power' (Heraud, 1973: 89), occupational therapy would be aligning itself with a marginalized group. It would be using its mandate to generate knowledge and its positional power in the interests of the disempowered.

All forms of understanding are culturally embedded constructions and are subject to challenge and change. Our 'knowledge' can be seen as a product of the social purposes and practices of time and place (Rorty, 1999). Policy reflecting the affirmative model would represent a challenge to the dominant biomedical discourse and offer an alternative to what Foucault (1980) calls a 'regime of truth'. Essentially this is the idea that societies, at different times in their historical development, produce sets of ideas that are imbued with the quality of 'truth'. The current 'regimes of truth' or ways of understanding are represented by the individual and tragedy models of disability. They have become part of our commonsense ways of understanding the world through the consistent reinforcement of learned definitions of reality (Berger and Luckmann, 1984).

From a socio-political perspective the involvement of disabled people and their representative organizations in the development of policy would also represent a shift away from a client model (Beresford and Croft, 1986) where users of services are marginalized within the organization and practice of caring professions. It would symbolize a move towards a citizenship model (Croft and Beresford, 1989; Taylor, 1989) where users of professional services are involved in the control of those services and, perhaps more radically, the production of knowledge informing them. A move towards a citizenship model would be a significant development for the profession. Kymlicka argues that 'liberal-democratic states should not only uphold the familiar set of common civil and political rights of citizenship which are protected in all liberal democracies; *they must also adopt various group-specific rights or policies which are intended to recognise and accommodate the distinctive identities and needs of ethocultural groups'* (2001: 42). Although Kymlicka argues from a macro state perspective, the fundamental idea of citizenship is equally applicable at an institutional or organizational level. The development of policy reflecting the affirmative model in alliance with disabled people has the potential to contribute to the creation of a social vision and aid the profession in the process of redefining its role, function and purpose.

Provision

Occupational therapists are predominantly employed within the National Health Service and local authority social care services throughout the UK. Their location in these service systems will pose genuine challenges to therapists attempting to use the affirmative model to inform service provision. The culture of the organization in which they work shapes and influences the ways in which occupational therapists define their role and structures the ways in which they provide a service. It can be argued that entry to the service system is dependent upon a defined problem or perceived deficit. The dynamic of the service system is based upon solving the problem or remediating the deficit. McKnight states that,

> while most professionals will agree that individual problems develop in a socio-economic–political context, their common remedial practice isolates the individual from context. The effect of this individualization leads the professional to distort even his own contextual understanding. Because his remedial tools and techniques are usually limited to individualized interaction, the interpretation of need necessarily becomes individualized. The tool defines the problem rather than the problem defining the tool. (1995: 43)

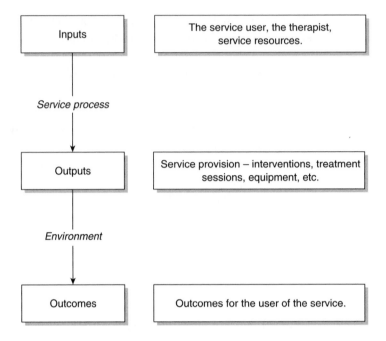

Figure 12.1   *The production of welfare model*

Thus occupational therapists will find a tension between the dynamic driving service provision, which is essentially individualized and problem based, and a view of impairment and disability as integral positive elements of a person's personal and collective identity.

The adoption of the affirmative model has another fundamental implication for current forms of occupational therapy service provision. The affirmative model will, by implication, challenge therapists to redefine their concept of the service users. A redefinition of service users, acknowledging positive elements of their experience of impairment and disability and locating them within a social context, will lead therapists to refocus their service provision. 'The production of welfare model', adapted from Davies and Knapp (1981), illustrates the relationship between what therapists think, what they provide and what happens for users of the service.

This model illustrates the way in which a change in inputs (affirmation model) will affect outputs (service provision), which in turn will influence outcomes for the users of the service. In practical terms it can be seen that what the therapist and the service user bring to the input stage will affect outcomes. Thus a change in the way in which occupational therapists conceptualize impairment and disability (input) will affect the nature of their service provision (output), which in turn will influence the outcome for the users of the service.

The lexicon of service provision has the potential to expand from diagnosis, assessment, treatment and intervention to include ideas of occupational justice (Townsend and Wilcock, 2004), occupational apartheid (Kronenberg and Pollard, 2005), rights, opportunities, choice and inclusion.

Practice

Wilcock (2000) has argued that a reductionist medical model has dominated the profession's way of viewing clients and their difficulties. The reductionist medical model focuses occupational therapy practice on the individuals' impairment and results in their experiences being pathologized. Hammel is sceptical of the uncritical way occupational therapists have embraced the World Health Organization's system of classifying disability and impairment. She advocates that: 'the assumptions, theories and practices of our profession should all be subjected to the type of skeptical analysis enabled by engagement with the work of critical disability theorists' (2004: 410). The current dominance of the medical model within practice is a key factor limiting occupational therapy practice. Given that disabled people may also have medical needs, the key challenge for OTs is to incorporate both the medical and the affirmative models into their practice.

Ideas of a partnership, client-centredness, enablement, empowerment and social inclusion are common in occupational therapy literature (Townsend, 1993; Baum and Christianson, 1997; Townsend and Brintell, 1997; Sumison, 1999; Kronenberg and Pollard, 2005). In theory, occupational therapy has a philosophical base that is potentially congruent with the affirmative model of disability. However, Kronenberg and Pollard have identified a theory/practice divide:

> a constructively critical look at everyday practice reveals a dissonance between our proclaimed philosophical roots, values and beliefs – who we say we are and what we stand for, our rhetoric – and what we do in practice in the real world, in relation to the people we serve. (2005: 63)

This dissonance between rhetoric and practice has been criticized both by OTs and by some outside the profession. Abberley is critical of the rhetoric of partnership and the holistic approach employed by occupational therapists. He states that, 'far from incorporating a social model of disability, Occupational Therapy's stance of voluntarism and holism constitutes a professional ideology in conflict with it' (1995: 231). Wright and Rowe argue that with the limited exception of Barber (2002) who developed a client-led referral system in an acute setting: 'the profession has opted to stress the apolitical notion of client-centred practice rather than the more robust challenges of service user involvement' (2005: 45).

Townsend suggests that the dissonance between the philosophy of client-centred theory and practice relates to the issues of power and justice that exist for clients and occupational therapists:

> Questions about power and justice are often viewed skeptically as being too political. Yet not addressing power and justice is also political; we can either remain silently compliant with client/consumer injustices and our professional lack of empowerment, or we can take a visible, active stance to advocate for change. (2004: 85)

The issues of identity and power are challenges to occupational therapy adopting an affirmative model and involving disabled people in shaping practice. Goren (2002) describes occupational therapy as youthful, unsure of its identity and sensitive to its environment. He optimistically presents this youthfulness as an opportunity to develop a more sensitive and mature way of working with clients. Moccelin (1996) suggests that the absence of a single convincing source of leadership and ideas to facilitate homogeneity is at the root of the profession's confusion, identity crisis and fragmentation. Laing, as cited in Thompson, describes the concept of ontological insecurity that may resonate with the profession's current identity, leading to inaction:

> In an external environment full of changes the person is obsessively preoccupied with apprehensions of possible risks to his or her existence and is paralyzed in terms of practical action. (2003: 30)

Some practitioners may find security in homogeneity, an evidence base and occupation-focused models. However, the profession should be cautious of addressing this professional insecurity by the over-rigid identification with positivist norms that exclude the narratives and expertise of disabled people. Occupational therapy needs to move away from a view that it is an end in itself, to a view of itself developing in partnership with disabled people. Thus its security will come from a clear view of the role it has in relation to engaging with disabled people as partners working for social and political change.

On a personal and interpersonal level there is a challenge for therapists to explore their own attitudes and values about impairment and disability. Townsend from a Canadian perspective quotes Jean-Pierre Galipeault, former owner of Empowerment Connection, a consulting business that provides mental health promotion strategies:

> If occupational therapists philosophically view consumers or survivors as they do any other member of society as having assets, capabilities and gifts that they bring to their communities, the focus will be taken off needs and the relationship

between customer and therapist will be built on hope, trust, strengths and equal participation. (2004: 79)

Sinclair, advocating a wider perspective on practice, suggests that:

Occupational therapists must develop their roles as agents of social change, taking the profession to a new level that makes a difference to entire communities as well as to the individuals we treat and encourage. To enable them to become effective agents of change the way in which occupational therapists are educated must come under sweeping review. (2005: xiv)

The incorporation of the affirmative model of disability into their practice has the potential to enable therapists to move away from predominantly individually focused interventions (McKnight, 1995) where provision is shaped by the available resources within their control. This is not to argue that people do not have individual needs that are most appropriately met on the individual level. It suggests that the affirmative model opens up possibilities for practice where the individual is understood as being located within a social context and that different outcomes then become possible.

Conclusion

Professional policy, provision and practice can be seen as inextricably interlinked. It is acknowledged that occupational therapy is a complex intervention often bridging the health and social care divide. It is often located at the interface between a person's medical needs and issues that are essentially socio-political in nature. The incorporation of an affirmative model of disability and impairment presents challenges to occupational therapy at every level. A key challenge will be to move away from an essentialist individual view of disabled people to one that locates them in a wider social context. It will also offer opportunities for the profession to develop new ways of working which genuinely affirm the experiences of disabled people and which reflect their hopes and aspirations as fellow citizens.

13 In Practice from the Viewpoint of a Physiotherapist

Anna-Stina with Sally French and John Swain

A different approach was taken in the writing of this chapter. It is based on the views of a physiotherapist, Anna-Stina, who wished to contribute to the book through being interviewed rather than writing the chapter herself. We complied with her wishes and this chapter is written from the transcript of an interview. Anna-Stina has worked for over thirty years as a physiotherapist: for the first twenty years in paediatrics; then the following ten years with adults with physical disabilities; and, at the time of the interview, with adults with profound and multiple impairments. The following then is her account of the development of her practice and thinking as a physiotherapist. It can be seen as a gradual progression within therapy practice towards a recognition of an affirmative model of disability and impairment and the challenges that such a redirection entails.

Anna-Stina's experiences and views

Anna-Stina began her career in a residential hospital for young people with multiple impairments, cerebral palsy and also cystic fibrosis. She told us:

> It was a case of giving these people treatment and you took them into a gym and they would be treated there, people with cerebral palsy would be positioned. It was also a surgical unit so I was involved in pre- and post-surgery, things like elongation of Achilles tendons, adductor tenotomies, hamstring releases and scoliosis. The chest physiotherapist took up hours which doesn't happen now,

we moved on from there. Every day every patient, as they were called then, had a morning session and an afternoon session, some of them had four or five sessions a day. We did percussion and breathing exercises for half an hour. The thing was to try and get them to produce mucus and that was success. It was analyzed and measured.

What were the attitudes of people to the disabled children? What was the philosophy of the place? How were they viewed?

It's very difficult for me to think in terms of how other people viewed them. If I reflect on it I suppose they, the 'patients', they were there to be treated. They were there for treatment and any thought about integrating this treatment into a daily life wasn't there. Their schooling came second. The sort of things that we talk about today with physiotherapy being part of life didn't happen then. Yes, we were there to treat the children, that was our job, they were being 'done to'.

Did they have parents who came to see them?

Yes, they had parents who came to visit and I suppose Tadworth was quite progressive in that they provided, as the years moved on, accommodation for parents. But the kids were away from home, they were just there. They lived there but they also came in for intensive periods. It was a respite centre as well. It was very much the doctors who ruled the roost.

Was education less of a priority?

There were teachers there and they were not prioritized as staff. It was the physiotherapists and the medical staff who were in charge and the teachers had to ask very kindly if they could possibly have access to the patients because the medical work was viewed as being so much more important. It was really prioritized. The teachers had to knock on the door gingerly and try and negotiate a time which would be suitable for a little bit of reading. Education was not prioritized, nor any other needs. If you look at activities of daily living or play, they didn't feature much. Staff tried to make the stay there as pleasant as possible, and there was play, but I don't know how much freedom there was.

What was the overall aim?

The aim was to get them 'better', to improve their medical condition. I can remember thinking that these people had other needs, but ideas of being client centred weren't around much. It was my own thoughts that I was battling with.

There may have been wishes that they had which could have been developed,
but such considerations weren't terribly prevalent.

Were the children involved in any decisions?

I can't imagine that they were. They were passive. That's how I perceive it. At that
time we put the callipers on and they had to walk. We know now that most of these
young people elect, when they're teenagers, to use wheelchairs instead of callipers
and walking aids but at that time mobility, in a broad sense, was not on the agenda.
It was walking, it was making them 'normal', that's what we strived for.

Did the children protest?

Yes, they didn't like it. They were not easy sessions and I didn't particularly enjoy
them either. I was a very junior physiotherapist and you're not allowed to … well
it was difficult for me to be assertive but there were some treatments that I didn't
enjoy doing at all.

Were they painful?

Yes, yes they were painful. With some of the surgical treatments we had to do
stretchings afterwards, which I questioned at the time but I didn't quite know how
to deal with it. Looking back there was this vast over-emphasis on medical needs
and we ignored other needs. I do feel we've moved on and looking at the whole
person has got to be the right answer. Their care needs were sorted, things like
bowels and continence and eating, whereas I feel where I am now I'm not so sure
that these needs are being cared for. I certainly think that the nursing care was
superb but we didn't look at the whole person in those days.

What did you do next?

I moved on because the hospital was about to close. I then worked in the
community. So for three years I worked in the community with the same client
group. Then I had contact with schools and I had contact with parents and that
was such an eye-opener for me.

How did it change the way you worked?

Well, I'd given exercise schemes to children in the hospital and when I looked at
the conditions that some of these children lived in and the burden that the
mothers had with looking after the children and their daily care, I thought 'there's
no way that this mum will be able to do these exercises.'

Also going into the schools, some of the schools were special schools and some of the schools had a class for disabled people and there was one school where a little boy with spina bifida was integrated. So I had the whole range there. Integration very much depended on the head. There was one super school where the head was brilliant. He had a holistic view. Another school allocated a bench and three hours on a Monday morning for me to do physiotherapy … I don't know what he expected me to do. Some of these kids needed climbing frames and big balls and all I had was this bench. It was such a battle and I had to bring in my supervisors. I needed access to the gym. I don't know what he thought physiotherapy was all about.

So, in a way, you lost status when you moved out of the hospital?

Yes. I also really questioned what I was doing, how I was contributing to these people's lives. Again it was looking after callipers and boots, but I questioned the value of my input. I don't think we questioned things to the extent that we do today. There was no evidence-based medicine then.

How did you find working with the parents?

I thought the parents were amazing, fantastic, but they had the problem of all these professionals coming to their homes that they had to look after and make coffee for. It was before key workers. These poor parents just had to be available and they didn't have a life of their own. Most of them went along with the advice as best they could. They were keen to do their best for the children and they took advice from the professionals.

So you moved on?

Yes, I'd heard about a Mobility Centre, we'd had some contact with them because some of our patients had needed electric wheelchairs and we didn't know enough about how to assess. It was something very tangible. To be able to assist and enhance somebody's mobility seemed to me to be just great. It was to do with any kind of outdoor mobility: manual wheelchairs, electric wheelchairs, scooters and driving assessments. Compared to the paediatric work this was much more focused and definite. It got away from an emphasis on walking. Some people were stuck at home so the idea of somebody driving a car was brilliant. Our role was to find solutions. There was a mixture of physiotherapists and OTs so there was good teamwork. It was very exciting. The OTs and physiotherapists complemented each other. We were trained as mobility therapists. We didn't treat people. We assessed what ability they had and how to compensate with adaptations which then made them mobile. Choice of vehicle is very important.

Did the disabled people have more involvement?

Yes, absolutely. The assessment was really an interview. Driving is such a motivator. The people who came had decided themselves, they'd made their own choice, they weren't sent by doctors, nobody told them to go there. They had their own ideas, they were prepared and they had thought about driving. Also their families were invited to the interviews. A partner may have a very valuable input. We were presented with a problem and it could be something as simple as getting an automatic car, or a two-door car, it was identifying what the barrier was and finding a solution to it. For people who had physical problems there was nearly always a solution but for people who had cognitive difficulties they were either borderline or it really wasn't possible, it wasn't safe.

Did you have doctors in the establishment?

We did, we had a doctor, a psychologist, an orthoptist, physiotherapists and OTs and a driving instructor. Today there are only physiotherapists and OTs and a driving instructor there.

Could you tell me a bit about your present job?

Things have changed tremendously because I'm now employed by a College of Further Education for students who are adults, over 19. It's a day college and, because it's run by teachers, the principal is a teacher and my manager is a teacher, it's very much an educationally based environment and medical needs come second. It's reversed so now I come and knock on the door and say, 'Please can I look at somebody and see what needs they may have?' I think that the strength of this, if you look at a person and call them a student instead of a patient and call the establishment a college instead of a day centre, is that it's much more empowering.

Is it difficult? Do you feel that you are at the bottom of the hierarchy?

I certainly have felt that way. I felt that way when I came into college one day and there was going to be an inspection and all the standing frames had disappeared. They didn't want such things to be around when these people came. They didn't want any medical evidence around.

It sounds less medicalized. Is this good? Are there disadvantages? What are your views?

I think the weakness is that, in my opinion and my experience, that basic medical and nursing needs are not met. The staff that work there are teachers and they are not medically trained and I do feel that it's important for students to be comfortable, basic needs like bowel management, sitting posture and monitoring of medication, but because the students are there to be taught it's not focused on in the same way. There's a holistic attitude and I believe that these things will be addressed, it's a new establishment, they're developing. A good thing about the college is that it's in the centre of a small town so Sainsbury's is across the road, the library is behind us. Students can go for a coffee, they can get on the bus, they can use local facilities: it's really integrated into the community and I like that. I find it very positive. That's a real strength. I feel confident that we'll move towards these issues that need to be developed. The staff are very motivated and open. There isn't that institutional background. We're creating something new here together.

We need to look at what each individual student needs and approach it from a client-centred point of view. We need to look at the networks of the student, the context and to draw on the people who are involved with the students. Things have improved vastly. There's a lot of fun and laughter, a lot of dance and music. It's my impression that this is what the students enjoy: many of them are not able to speak but you can see it in their facial expressions.

How much of an input do they have as to what goes on? Are they consulted?

Yes, a consensus is needed for whatever we do, so if there is something that they don't want to do, say a physiotherapy treatment, they have a choice of saying 'no'. That takes the pressure off the physiotherapy. We're here to support the teachers so that the full potential of the student is being achieved. The physiotherapist is now much more integrated so instead of me giving a session in the gym, the person walks to the toilet, instead of doing passive movements on a mat they'll be done when the person's pad is being changed. It's woven into the activities of the day. Standing in the standing frame might be done during the music session. They're not standing in the standing frame because that's what the physiotherapist wants them to do, they're standing in the standing frame so that they can do something like learning to play an instrument or use a computer.

Conclusion

At the end of her interview Anna-Stina provided a very apt conclusion to this chapter. She told us:

I think I've learned far more from all the people than they've learned from me.

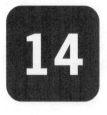

Communication Disability: Exploring New Personal and Professional Narratives

Carole Pound

In recent years increasing attention has been paid to practical ways of applying social model principles to professional practice in speech and language therapy (SLT). This is echoed in a small but growing literature from academics, practitioners and innovators who write about personal and professional struggles to institute social model practices and attend practically to the values that underpin new ways of working (Pound, 2004; Byng and Duchan, 2005; Swinburn, 2005; van der Gaag and Mowles, 2005).

Many speech and language therapists have also taken seriously government and professional body mandates to involve service users more widely and authentically in decision making and the planning of more user-focused services. There are increasing examples of good practice where people with communication impairment are involved as teachers, writers, researchers, evaluators, policy advisors and, in some cases, deliverers of services (Byng and Duchan, 2005; Hewerdine and Laugesen,2005; Duchan, 2006).

In addition, a growing number of interventions address barriers to participation and the role of the speech and language therapist and others in removing these barriers. Thus, rather than expending precious resources predominantly on impairment-focused assessments and remediating the impaired communication skills of the individual, practitioners are beginning to consider whether best value relates more pertinently to changing the communication skills of conversational partners and attending to inaccessible communication environments. For example Kagan (1998) and others have long advocated training for conversational partners such as spouses so that they can converse better with people with acquired communication impairments. Parr et al. (in press) also promote ways to enhance communication access to health and social care services.

It is clear therefore that there has been some progress in shifting the focus and philosophy of intervention. Social model principles, practices and language are becoming more familiar in the world of speech and language therapy. However, with this greater awareness has come a sharper focus on the persisting barriers to change. This chapter will draw on conversations with people living with long-term communication disability and the practitioners who work with them to illustrate some of the key challenges to equalizing relationships and power. It will give examples of practical approaches to operating within a non-tragedy view of acquired communication impairment and suggest options for the next steps towards engaging with an affirmative model of disability.

Barriers to progress

Connect has offered training courses for practitioners working in the area of stroke care. The courses on social model practice in medical model settings highlight a range of barriers to adopting more social model principles in Connect's work. Connect is a national charity working to promote effective services, new opportunities and a better quality of life for people living with aphasia (http://www.ukconnect.org/). Some of the ways of addressing barriers to change include having the group problem-solve about how to:

- manage patients' and relatives' firmly held expectations of recovery and cure;
- balance efforts to operate person-centred practices within systems-driven organizations;
- address temporal barriers to more inclusive practices, for example finding the time to make information and the process of information sharing accessible to people with communication impairments (Pound and Hewitt, 2004);
- recognize personal and professional insecurity about straying from the role and interventions defined in therapist/training;
- work towards team sharing of a value system in spite of the hurly-burly of everyday service delivery;
- tone down powerful and dominant professional voices within the team that may disempower both staff members and patients. For example, it can be hard to make your voice heard on a ward round if you feel you lack the power and status to do so;

- contend with feelings of powerlessness at the thought of changing and challenging deeply embedded cultures involving language and rituals that sustain professional power.

Whilst these barriers often seemed most marked for those working within the strict professional hierarchies and entrenched routines of acute medical settings, they also exist for practitioners in community settings and home-based services.

Why do some of these hurdles feel so insurmountable, particularly given, at one level, the willingness of practitioners to enhance their services through quality listening, authentic partnerships and 'empowerment' focused goals? What are the cultural underpinnings of professional practice that sustain and defend traditional divisions between professional power and user control? A short, but by no means exhaustive list might include the following systemic sources of difficulty.

Training

Many training colleges now include disability equality training and attend explicitly to the social model of disability within the core curriculum. Stories and talks by those who live with a communication impairment pepper lectures about different impairments and the everyday impact of conditions on lives. And slowly, but increasingly, there is a literature and new 'evidence base' of disabled people's own narratives on which to build student knowledge (Parr et al., 2003). There is widespread recognition that it is the first-hand stories of people who live the inside experience that will have the most lasting impact on students.

However, the absence of people with communication impairment on the staff or in other positions of power, for example planning the curriculum, accrediting courses, informing professional bodies or indeed having access to academic debates within university departments and professional bodies, suggests that there is some way to go.

Despite some attempts to reconfigure the curriculum to place greater emphasis on the social construction and impact of different conditions, many courses remain aetiology led, privileging the professional expertise required to manage conditions resulting in communication impairment. So whilst van der Gaag and Anderson (2005) identify positive patterns of change in the outlook of new SLT graduates, they also note the continuing preference of newly qualified speech and language therapists to project themselves as experts.

Polarization, simplification and the social model muddle

Recently therapists have been engaged in discussions about the relative benefits of social model or impairment focused approaches to intervention. This reductionistic dichotomy is manifested for example in conferences on aphasia where linguistic, deficit-based approaches run in parallel sessions to more social approaches to intervention. It is apparent when therapists talk about juggling their time between: (1) supporting people with communication impairments to address real social needs and barriers; and (2) making the best use of hard-won specialist knowledge and ways to enhance their service users' communicative independence. This divide falsely reduces the complex social relations of therapy and the breadth of therapeutic possibilities to an either/or therapeutic approach reflecting, it seems, the tendency within the therapy professions to assert professional power through a polarization of approaches to therapy.

Byng and Duchan (2005) have criticized and explored this polarization in relation to interventions for and with people who have aphasia. They argued that the discussion should not be whether a therapy is of a 'social model type' or an 'impairment model type' but about how therapists interact with people who have aphasia. How are choices and decisions made? Who is accountable to whom? What range of roles can the person with aphasia and the therapist take rather than remaining trapped in the expert therapist/impaired patient dyad? Social model practices call on us not just to think about the type of therapy we are doing but, crucially, about the way expertise, accountability and power sharing underpin the therapeutic endeavour.

Additionally, there is some confusion resulting from a misunderstanding that socially orientated goals are synonymous with social model practices. For example, many clinicians associate work on 'functional, practical activities', such as learning to use the phone or how to use money when buying a bus ticket, with disability-type therapies. The intervention continues to focus on the skills and achievements of the communication-impaired individual, however, rather than on the disabling communication practices of others and the communicatively inaccessible environment around them. Whilst many therapists acknowledge their role as advocate, social campaigner and agent of social change, these aspects of therapist identity remain less comfortable and less familiar territory than the one-to-one interactions focussing on skill acquisition, building personal independence or supporting communication-impaired individuals to grieve for lost abilities.

Interactions and report writing – the discourse of incompetence

Researchers who have examined the discourse of therapeutic interactions have discovered how disempowering clinical interactions can be. Simmons-Mackie and Damico (1999) have studied the talking patterns in a typical therapy session. First the therapist elicits a piece of known information, for example asking what something is called. Second the client responds with their answer. Third the therapist evaluates the client's response for its proximity to the required target. This 'therapy dance' not only reinforces the powerful role of competent helper evaluating incompetent client but echoes the discourse patterns used in other authority-based hierarchies such as courtrooms (Panagos, 1996) and the traditional classroom.

Addressing the language of incompetence, Duchan (1999) also highlights the cultural practice of report writing that plays to the deficit model of communication, locating the problem firmly with the impaired person.

Cultural narratives of disability – the stronghold of heroes and victims

Discussion about cultural representations of disability have begun to surface. There are debates among professionals about how language and images promote or challenge traditional negative stereotyping of disabled people. Within social care, the voluntary sector and to some extent healthcare, service providers are increasingly aware that the language and discourse of biomedicine may not always be the most appropriate language to use when referring to disabled people, particularly when they are many years into a life with a disabling condition. But the infantilizing and problematizing vocabulary of 'patients', 'sufferers', 'assessment', 'referral' and 'discharge' remains the common currency of much service provision. Those who have few words and little voice are thus trapped within the perpetual passivity of the patient world. Taking control and being an equal citizen require that a more active and respectful vocabulary and grammar be used both by those who live with a communication disability and, crucially, by those who provide services to them.

Speech and language therapists have a particular interest in language and some therapists in recent years have paid greater attention to the language and vocabulary of disability. Like many health and social care workers they are now more aware of the impact of labelling. So one no longer finds references in clinical discourse to people as aphasics, dysarthrics, MS sufferers and stroke victims. Within day-to-day practice there are determined attempts to model change in the language of reports, leaflets and information for service users.

However, the changes needed to achieve affirmative models of disability clearly go beyond words. Hero and victim narratives are alive and well in the minds and attitudes of service providers and emerge in a range of ways. Two such examples that are regularly encountered within our own training programme are: (1) service provider reactions to our use of disabled people as teachers; and (2) service provider reactions to affirming statements by disabled people.

Key words on feedback forms continue to make reference to how 'brave' the speaker was to stand up and speak, or what an 'inspiration' they are to others. Responses to disabled teachers as heroes rather than as providers of information are indicated in levels of applause and lack of challenge. Chris Ireland, who lives with aphasia, penned the ironic 'Creative Window Truthteller' poem (unpublished, 1999). As the following extract illustrates, the challenge for practitioners is not to treat speakers with language impairments as heroes or victims but as partners in creativity:

No heroes, no victims

No worship, no patients

No workshirt, no villains

No workshirkers, but pigeon poetry power

No horseshit, but by seeking philospher stone.

Not labels, but as artists and scientists explorers,

Each, through own creative windows,

Breath of fresh air reflecting

Working together for new creative ramps.

Another interesting litmus test for disabling discourse is the audience reaction to a disabled person who states unequivocally that their life is better and more enriched since their disability. For many practitioners such statements can only be comprehended as a manifestation of at best poor judgement and at worst lack of insight on the part of the person expressing them. Moreover, ensuing discussions frequently raise passionate defences of known clients who unequivocally portray themselves as an impaired sufferer and depleted individual. This, they argue, is a reality not to be diminished by the politics of disability.

Therein it seems lies the real challenge for many practitioners – to widen their understanding of disability and the range of responses of different individuals without feeling the need to operate an either/or approach. For some practitioners the social model of disability is at least a left field option but the affirmative orientation to disability may not yet be in the ballpark.

Engaging with access and affirmation

What then are some of the practical ways practitioners can extend their repertoire of services and support to build on these advances in awareness and intent? What might clinicians and managers do to systematically redirect precious resources and energy in favour of promoting more equal relations between service providers and their language-disabled clients? Below are some ideas drawn from our own practice at Connect. We actively espouse collaboration, power sharing and the possibility for all people with aphasia to connect with the affirmative model of disability. At the same time, we acknowledge the challenges facing us in a world where language is power, where society is still dominated by the grand narrative of impairment as deficit and where organizations are founded and led by professionally trained clinicians and academics who are imbued with the impairment paradigm.

Promoting the affirmative model of disability within professional practice – Ideas from Connect

1 Identify the key sources of power and decision making within the organization and seek to place people who live with communication impairment in key positions – as members of staff, as researchers, as project managers and as advisors and activists. Ensure that appropriate resources and infrastructure are in place to enable people to fulfil these roles. For example, extra time is needed to line-manage employees with communication impairment, and to attend pre and post meetings to enable advisors with language impairments to fully understand and rehearse the strategic issues and information under discussion.

2 Support disabled people not just to feed into consultations but to take leadership roles in planning and delivering services. This might also include ensuring that people are involved in and share responsibility for difficult decisions about prioritizing resources or identifying criteria for rationing services.

3 Ensure that the organization models and embodies difference in a tangible way, such as by having communicatively accessible environments and documents, people with communication impairments who are acknowledged leaders and experts, or people with aphasia who openly celebrate their aphasia and their life as an aphasic person.

4 Support non-disabled staff and volunteers to discuss, reflect on and challenge their own attitudes and understanding of disability, both within mandatory disability equality training but also on an ongoing basis. For example reflections and feedback on establishing and maintaining more equal relationships with communication-impaired people can be integrated into 360 degree appraisal systems, performance management and the organizational review of standards.

5 Establish and monitor clear standards of communication access in the conversations that take place in your workplace, the documents and information you produce and the way your environment supports or impedes communicating differently. Ensure that all staff (professional, clerical, volunteers) have training in communication access in the same way that all staff will undergo manual handling or fire training.

6 Make sure attention to communication access and skills in making interactions, events, meetings, documents and environments communicatively accessible is an issue shared by everyone in your organization rather than just the very few.

7 Encourage access to personal and local support when challenging dominant medicalized cultures, routines and rituals. For example extra time is needed to reflect and plan, reassurance and support are needed to persevere when an initiative hits a problem, and supervision is needed to reflect on long-term benefits for service users or ways to bolster confidence and self-esteem when relinquishing power.

8   Ensure that alternative narratives of disability are surfaced, shared and listened to. For example, support disabled people who are engaging in the creation of publications and websites, and in everyday workplace interactions.

9   Attend to culture, values and philosophy of practice with the same attention as is traditionally placed on systems and outcomes.

Conclusion

Increasingly, speech and language therapists are recognizing that sharing power is not something to be merely espoused in role play or as an 'empowerment' technique. Rather it is a critical part of improving services and making them relevant to the lives of people who live with a communication impairment. This is no longer a choice but an imperative. There are encouraging signs of reflection on the requirement to work differently, translating sometimes into changed awareness and sometimes changed action. Progress towards a more equal relationship between speech and language therapists and people with communication impairment seems for most to require engagement with a three-stage process: adopting the language of the social model but retaining the goal of 'functional independence' as the driving force behind therapy; engaging both intellectually and practically with social model principles while retaining most of the power; and understanding and embracing the true challenge of walking the affirmative model walk. As the examples and accounts of different ways of working together increase, hopefully there will be a growing confidence to take the next step towards the affirmative model of disability.

15 In Practice from the Viewpoint of a Disabled Nurse

Rachael Spain

It is a sad fact that, even today, at the beginning of the twenty-first century, more than a decade after the Disability Discrimination Act was passed, the predominant model of disability still revolves around the medical model, with its focus on impairments rather than people. This model emphasizes the search for a cure, and has cast medical personnel in the role of 'experts'. The medical model is also overlaid by the tragedy model in the minds of these medically orientated personnel, as they are the gatekeepers of so many of the resources which disabled people require. Recently though, doctors and nurses are beginning to admit that they are definitely not experts on disability and disability issues. This is borne out by work, done over three years and culminating in 2005 in the report 'Different Differences: disability equality teaching in healthcare education', by Bristol University, the University of the West of England and the Peninsula Medical School. The work pioneers the incorporation of disability equality into training for medical students and nurses and also incorporates disabled people as active contributors. This is the first step on the long road towards seeing disabled people as equal human beings.

Given that traditionally the healthcare system has such a negative approach to disabled people, what happens to a disabled person who wishes to become a nurse? How is the nursing profession going to accept a disabled person as 'fit to practise'? Nursing is seen as such a physically active role, and one that involves such a significant amount of patient contact, that even the terminology of 'fit to practise' gives the impression of being robustly able-bodied. How can people who have qualified as nurses and then become disabled carry on with such a career? Nursing is supposed to cure people, and return them to former health again. So how can a disabled person, for whom there is no apparent cure, be allowed to play a role in helping other patients to be cured?

The barriers for disabled nurses: training

It is against this subconscious background of beliefs that disabled people have to battle to be allowed to gain admission to nurse training and/or continue within the nursing profession. They have to negotiate themselves into a position where members of this profession will recognize, and accept, them as colleagues. They will also have to cope with the possibility that society needs time to adjust and not be alarmed at having a disabled nurse in a caring role rather than as seen through the usual perception of a disabled person needing, not giving, care.

There are two main strands that need to be considered, one being disabled people who wish to train to become nurses; and the other the nurse who acquires an impairment having been already registered as a nurse. A further issue that will affect career aspirations will be the nature of the impairment and whether it is hidden or obvious.

Taking, first, the possibilities of training as a nurse if a person is disabled, the main issue will probably be the nature of the impairment. In the United Kingdom, the hidden impairment of dyslexia, for example, would not necessarily preclude a person from undertaking a nursing training and there are a significant number of students who, with specialist support, are both in training and have qualified as nurses (Wright, 2000). This is, however, a recent development.

The Nursing and Midwifery Council (NMC), which is the regulatory body of the nursing profession, requires that all students demonstrate their 'fitness to practise' at the end of their training, before they are admitted to the register and can call themselves a nurse.

> In order to register applicants have to declare and have confirmed by the leader of their programme that they are in good health and character sufficient to ensure safe and effective care. The NMC believes that, whilst it may be possible for an individual with a health problem/disability to achieve the stated competencies and be fit for practice on completion, it does not necessarily follow that the individual is subsequently employable in all fields of practice. (NMC, 2006: 1)

It also recommends that universities meet with students at the application stage, and that students are screened for any health issues that could affect their planned career.

Discussions about how the requirements could be met, through making 'reasonable adjustments' within the scope of the Act, enable both the potential applicant and the university to come to a realistic decision about progressing an application. Where the decision is to proceed with the application, the university will be expected to comply with their responsibilities under the Disability Discrimination Act and related Codes of Practice. Where it is decided not to proceed, the NMC would hope that the university could offer some career advice. (NMC, 2006: 2)

The determination of disabled people to enter this profession is evidenced by the growing number of disabled students applying for nursing training. Role models such as Victoria Eathorne, currently a disability nurse advisor for the Cornwall NHS Trust, who qualified over ten years ago, provide inspiration. She had a car accident when she was nine years old and decided that she desperately wanted to be a nurse. After significant effort she entered training in the late 1980s. She explained it was:

hard at times ... Because I was brain-damaged it affected my speech – it is still slightly slow – and I also have a tremor in my right hand that is exacerbated by stress ... I had to deal with negative attitudes. In a busy working environment when nurses are under stress and somebody is seen to be not as quick as them, there can be a lack of understanding. (Coombs, 2004)

In the USA there has been growing momentum to include disabled people in nursing training, spearheaded by Maheady (2003). She has written extensively, and her recommendations include drawing up a specific learning contract between each student and the education establishment outlining what is expected from each by the other. The contract is divided up into sections covering clinical areas, and academic areas, and the specialist equipment required and allowed. It is set out in document form, the contents being what the training establishment, the individual tutors and the individual themselves will undertake to try and minimize the effect that disability could have on both learning and practice, and this is signed by all parties. It also sets long-term and short-term goals, enabling the measurement of achievements. When the short-term goals are monitored on a regular basis, it can be used to identify any shortfalls or unforeseen requirements. This is proving popular in the USA, with a growing number of students, who have a wide variety of impairments (cerebral palsy, hearing loss and T4 paraplegia, to name but a few) completing nurse training and gaining employment.

Currently in the UK there is no such uniform approach. Nikki Heazell, who had her left arm amputated at the elbow as a baby, decided early on in her life that she wanted to be a nurse and no one was stopping her!

Careers advisors always told me I couldn't do nursing, as it needed 'dexterity', something that I didn't have. Outwardly I said, 'Ok then', but inwardly I was saying to myself 'well sod you'. Careers advisors always tried to deter me from nursing by advising that I go into health related subjects like health science or health studies.

I applied to do my degree at a few universities throughout the country. Following my initial applications, I received a letter from one particular university saying that I had to be rejected from the course as I was termed as 'unfit', due to my only having one hand and the 'physical dexterity' that the job entailed. They hadn't even seen me or seen what I could do!

I had never really thought of myself as having a disability; however my rejection and blatant discrimination from that one university kind of changed my thinking. I was more annoyed that they assumed that I couldn't do nursing before they had even seen me or seen what I could do. The rejection was not justified and I thought that if the university was going to be that narrow-minded, then I didn't want to attend it anyway. (Disability Rights Commission, 2003: 1)

Nikki Heazell trained six years ago. Since then the Special Educational Need and Disability Act 2001 (SENDA) has been passed, making it unlawful for higher educational establishments to discriminate against current or prospective students on the grounds of disability. This means that disabled individuals with a disability are more likely to be accepted for nurse and midwifery education than they were previously. Students who disclose their impairments are also eligible for a Disabled Student Allowance (Department of Education and Skills, 2005/06) which helps to cover some of the extra expenses that their studying incurs and will also mean that supportive measures are put into place by student services officers, who have specific responsibilities for disabled students with a disability. A snapshot of a random London university, through information gained from their disability support department, shows that in 2006 eight students with physical impairments were studying nursing, indicating that this move towards admitting disabled students to nursing courses is slowly taking place.

Nurses becoming disabled

What then of nurses who acquire an impairment once qualified? Here again there is a slow shift towards the possibility of these nurses being allowed to return to their rightful place in the workforce. The predominant picture is still one of nurses being 'retired' from their profession once they have acquired an impairment that impinges in any way on the 'fit' image of the 'healthy' nurse.

The pattern that emerges on talking to nurses, who have acquired an impairment, is that they feel totally discarded by the profession:

I was injured by a patient. My injuries required two operations and I was on sick leave for six months. I then received a letter telling me that it had been decided

> *that I was to be medically retired. I couldn't believe that a caring profession could be so callous. I felt a total failure, my whole life plan just wiped out and no way to appeal. (University of Bristol News, 2005)*

It is very difficult to deal with such rejection, to fight it, and to try and take up a place within the profession again. Culturally there is still a deep-seated belief, even amongst those nurses who are disabled themselves, that there is a need to be 'fit to practise'; that is they are totally convinced that the word 'fit' means physically whole as well as mentally able. It is difficult enough to cope with a newly acquired impairment, but also to have to cope with how the 'caring' profession now deals with a previous colleague in such a totally different way can mean that making adjustments to disability takes far longer. To be treated as a patient rather than a nurse also brings some unpalatable revelations:

> *It was as if my knowledge was wiped out along with my acquisition of the paraplegia. Treatment was decided for me and procedures were explained in minimal terms. If I asked for more participation in my care it was dismissed as if it was too complicated for me to understand. This treatment eroded and then destroyed my self-confidence. (University of Bristol News, 2005)*

Similar experiences are recounted by Maheady (2006).

Disabled nurses: affirmation

There is now a dawning realization that nurses, who are disabled themselves, can offer rich insight into difficulties encountered by patients. Nikki Heazell, working competently as a nurse with one hand, states:

> *I do believe that my disability benefits my work. For example, I am able to show patients who have had a stroke and can only use one arm how to do things with one hand. Also, I find that I put a lot of mums at ease whose children have had a limb amputated, in particular their daughters. For example a lot of mums ask me how their daughters will put their bras on or shave under their arms. (DRC, 2003: 2)*

The Department of Health states the following guidance for the retention of health service employees:

> *Most disabled people become so during their working lives. By retaining someone who is disabled rather than letting them go, lets you keep their skill and experience and so avoid the cost and inconvenience of replacing them.*
>
> *Disabled people have as wide a range of talents as the rest of society. Some develop new skills in response to life as a disabled person, such as organizational skills from juggling care needs. These are often overlooked and good practice can help you capitalise on them.*

A representative workforce will enable you to relate with confidence to the needs and expectations of your patients and service users. Disabled people can help inform the development of good practice for patients, and working with disabled people can help other staff who work with disabled patients. (DoH, 2000: 14–15)

This document acknowledges the loss of valuable members of the workforce by simply retiring people who acquire a disability, which again is having an effect on the retention of disabled nurses.

WING (Work Injured Nurses Group) is a section within the Royal College of Nursing. Originally set up to support nurses who have been injured at work (predominantly back injuries), it now works with all member nurses who acquire an impairment, offering counselling, advice and small grants. It is currently working actively to encourage the employment of disabled nurses in all areas of the NHS and has produced supportive guidance in the form of 'Workability' documents (Royal College of Nursing, 2003).

This recognition that many disabled nurses have skills and experiences that are currently being wasted has also been made by newly developing areas of service. In the 'modern' NHS, many health services that were previously part of secondary care have been moved into primary care. This in turn has led to the development of new ways of working, for example the use of telephone triage as a method of assessing patients' care needs, which means that many patients can be competently dealt with by nurses. This has led to the creation of new roles that lend themselves to disabled nurses although it should not be expected that they work solely in these areas.

The development of NHS Direct, a national triage service, has written within its recruiting policy positive discrimination in terms of the employment of disabled nurses:

NHS Direct is a helpline service offered by the NHS to provide the public with the opportunity to obtain advice on health matters from qualified nurses …

All nurses recruited to NHS Direct in England will have to have attained the appropriate competencies and the recruitment of disabled nurses or those who have retired due to ill health is encouraged. (NHS Direct, 2006)

Changes are taking place all over the United Kingdom as the Disability Discrimination Act 1995, which was updated and strengthened by further legislation in 2005, has had an impact. NHS Trusts in both primary and secondary care have become more aware of the need to review their policies and their treatment of disabled people.

The Act sets out what is known as the General Duty. This means they will all have to have due regard to the need to eliminate unlawful discrimination and promote equal opportunities for disabled people. They will also need to consider the elimination of harassment of disabled people, promotion of positive attitudes and

the need to encourage the participation of disabled people in public life.
(Disability Rights Commission, 2005: 2)

Disabled nurses, and particularly those with management experience, have suddenly been seen as a useful commodity in drafting these policies and auditing their implementation:

> I am now regularly involved in a variety of roles with my local Primary Care Trust. My nursing background, coupled with the development of multiple long-term limiting conditions, makes me a useful member of the team as I bring not only patient perceptions, but an understanding of budgets and departmental/trust constraints, and an in-depth understanding of the physiology, pharmacology and other treatments of the conditions. I am involved with reviewing, and also regularly auditing the effectiveness of the Trust's anti-discriminatory policy, which includes spot check visits to see how I am treated as I am visually impaired and wheelchair dependent. This work has made all the difference, as I feel valued, but without the pressure when I have exacerbations of my conditions. (University of Bristol News, 2006)

Conclusion

The way forward is to move perception away from what a disabled person cannot do towards valuing them for what they can do. Their methods of adapting to society's demands and the environment can offer possible new insight into making the environment more accessible, and especially into ways of working with patients and for staff.

Because of advances in modern medicine, conditions that previously would have been fatal are now treatable to a point. Many conditions are not curable at present, but are manageable to the extent that these people can live a productive life within the parameters of their impairment. Impairment can happen to anyone, at any time of life.

It is reassuring that there is a slow, but significant, trend towards not just dismissing nurses because they are different but also accepting what they may do differently and valuing that difference and learning from it. There is hope for a future where it is commonplace to see nurses who are not the stereotypical 'whole-body perfection' working normally, especially in areas where their personal understanding can be of use, for example stroke units, but also throughout the entire health service.

16 In Practice from the Viewpoint of a Social Worker

Maureen Gillman

> *Diversity is starting to become a new 'buzz-word' ... The notion of valuing (or affirming or even celebrating) diversity relates to the idea that we should appreciate diversity as a positive factor, an asset rather than a problem to be solved. (Harrison et al., 2003: 7–8)*
>
> It is difficult to imagine any social worker, (or, for that matter, any health and social care professional,) admitting to *not* valuing diversity and difference. Indeed, such notions are claimed to be central to social work values of anti-oppressive practice and inclusive working (Dominelli, 1998; Humphries, 2004). However, whilst most practitioners would claim and genuinely believe that they adhere to such principles when working with disabled people, it is questionable to what extent such claims are merely rhetoric. This chapter reflects upon the issues raised in Chapter 11 and highlights the constraints and opportunities for social workers attempting to work collaboratively with disabled people in the current professional and policy contexts. The chapter ends with a reflection on the changes required at the various levels of context of professional social work.

Making distinctions to create connections

A distinction can be made between the values espoused by the social work profession and the dominant discourses, values and ideologies that shape many of the organizations that employ social workers. Social workers may leave their initial training courses with a commitment to the principles underpinning the social model of disability, but they will no doubt meet problems in putting these principles into practice in organizations dominated by the individual and biological models of disability. Although this distinction is often recognised by service users, in the literature professionals and their employing organisations are often referred to as if they were the same. Making a clearer distinction between professionals and their employers opens up options for change: for example the possibility of forming partnerships with disabled people which would not only benefit the service user but also provide support for the social worker wishing to promote more inclusive and collaborative practices in her organization. On this theme, Dominelli suggests that social workers may:

> adopt an openly political stance which can create complications between social workers' professional roles and their activities as social change agents. In this context, gaining the support of sympathetic others outside the social work remit is an important facet of the job. (1998: 5)

The social model and professional social work

Since the emergence of social work as a profession there has always been a tension between the notions of social reform and social control as legitimate activity for practitioners. These elements are reflected in social work training programmes which include such diverse subjects as structural inequalities, systemic and social constructionist approaches to change, counselling, and legal and managerial frameworks. Tensions about the direction that social work should take are reflected in all levels of the profession and compounded by the political and organizational contexts and drivers of the day.

Social model approaches to a variety of practice contexts such as mental health, ageing and disability, however, have long been regarded as the territory of the social work profession. Social model approaches are seen as one of the clear features distinguishing social work professionals from those who are members of professions allied to medicine in the health and social care arena. Jones et al. argue that

> More than any other Welfare State profession social work seeks to understand the links between 'public issues' and 'private troubles' and seeks to address both. It is for this reason that many who hold power and influence in our society would be delighted to see a demoralised and defeated social work, a social work that is incapable of drawing attention to the miseries and difficulties which beset so many in our society. (2006: 1)

Social model understanding and approaches are embedded within the curriculum of the new Social Work Degree (General Social Care Council, 2002) and the new Post-Qualifying Framework for Training and Education in Social Work (General Social Care Council, 2004).

Social model theory is translated into social work practice through the notion of anti-oppressive and inclusive practice that are claimed by the profession to be firmly embedded within professional identity and values. Social workers are expected to recognize and challenge structural inequalities associated with race, gender, religion, class, culture, sexuality, ability and age. In 1998, the social work academic, Dominelli, argued that those who engage in an emancipatory form of social work have an explicit commitment to social justice and to overtly challenging the welfare system. She went on to say that:

> Valuing 'difference' is one dimension of the complexities of life to be addressed explicitly by practitioners subscribing to anti-oppressive practice. (1998: 10)

Policy, provision and professional power

Recent policy developments such as service user involvement, direct payments and partnership working suggest that power imbalances between social care organizations and service users have been successfully addressed. On the surface, it would appear that such policy developments support the aspirations of social workers wishing to stay true to their professional values. The highest context marker in social care organizations, however, remains the bureaucratic and instrumental management of scarce resources. Social workers find themselves in the invidious and confusing position of having to use assessment instruments and criteria designed to limit the distribution of resources, yet cloaked in the rhetoric of empowerment, equity and partnership. Assessment criteria and instruments are steeped in the characteristics of the individual model of disability and informed by definitions such as those contained in the Disability Discrimination Act 1995.

Frameworks of assessment act as lenses or filters and dictate what can be taken into account and what should be ignored. Research with social workers employed in a social services adult care team (Swain et al., 1998) revealed that the emphasis on individual assessment had restricted activity such as the representation of the views of oppressed groups within the community. Furthermore, restrictions imposed by the assessment documentation, and rigid systems of prioritizing requests for assistance, have eroded their professional social work role and judgement.

In the 1960s and 1970s, social work was profoundly influenced by the anti-Vietnam War, Black and Women's movements (Jones et al., 2006). The 1970s witnessed the birth of the Radical Social Work Movement that placed the highest priority on the collective mobilization of groups, such as benefit claimants or council tenants, while rejecting the traditional casework approach for making clients 'come to terms' with unacceptable situations (Langan, 1998). Whilst the Radical Social Work movement itself is no longer in existence, many aspects of it have been integrated into mainstream practice, such as the inclusion of anti-racism and anti-sexism within the regulatory framework of social work values.

Despite social work's radical underpinnings (Bailey and Brake, 1975; Langan and Lee, 1989; Langan, 1998), developments in social work over the past ten years have weakened the impetus for social reform. Walton argues that

> *professional judgement is increasingly bound up with, and potentially subordinated*
> *by, managerial imperatives concerning corporate objectives and resource control.*
> *(2005: 596)*

The overriding concern of many social work managers is the control of budgets rather than the welfare of service users and this has created further distance between managers and front line workers (Jones et al., 2006).

Humphries argues that under New Labour social work has moved from a concern with welfare to a position of authoritarianism. She goes on to say that:

> *The practice of social work is increasingly perceived by Government as narrowly*
> *concerned with regulation and risk ... It has robbed social work of its radical and*
> *transformatory potential. (2004: 94)*

The concept of 'risk' and the practice of 'risk management' appear to have grown in importance in professional circles. Individuals are deemed to be at risk if their behaviour or circumstances is perceived by professionals as being a danger to themselves or others. This has implications for disabled people's encounters with professionals in relation to pursuing desired lifestyles that might be perceived under these criteria as risky or dangerous. Furthermore, protocols for assessing risk can be used to justify exclusion, incarceration and restraint. Beattie et al., writing about dementia care services, observe:

> *A further impact of the shift to community-based care has been a return to*
> *discourses of confinement, linked to notions of risk and dangerousness ... there*
> *are evident tensions between the felt or perceived needs of users and carers ...*
> *and prevalent concerns about security and risk, perhaps linked to notions of*
> *social order. (2005: 69)*

A central tenet of social work values is respecting and protecting the service user's right to self-determination. There is a delicate balance and tension between rights and risks in all cases, however, worked with by social workers. Maintaining such a balance has, in the past, been achieved by social workers using their professional judgement informed by social work values. Criticism of social workers in relation to their risk management in the contexts of, for example, child protection and the growth of the blame culture has resulted in the imposition of risk management procedures and protocols by their employers. This is another facet of risk management designed to protect professionals' backs. As one social worker recently put it, 'the highest context marker in managing risk is your own backside' (personal communication).

The notion of 'risk' organizes and shapes instruments of assessment and criteria for allocating scarce resources. Most local authority social services teams have developed a 'formula' for prioritizing requests for assistance. Banks and Williams conducted research on the issues, problems and dilemmas associated with ethical practice in social work. They describe the arrangements for prioritizing work in one local authority:

The assessment and information team is responsible for taking all new referrals to the department and screening them against eligibility criteria [which] had been relatively recently developed ... reflecting a growing preoccupation in social services generally with prioritizing and targeting resources at those most 'in need' or 'at risk', according to standardised criteria and matrices. (2005: 1014)

An example of the criteria is described by a social services manager:

Priority one represent a case where the situation has collapsed, or is about to collapse, and you are required to provide some kind of care package where they would be safe ... Priority two is a situation which is going to break down and should be dealt with, in theory, within two weeks. Cases that are priority one and two get done because they have to. Priority three cases are supposed to get dealt with in twenty days and it is where people could use some help; the classic is a case where assistance with bathing is needed ... We all accept that they need that but it is not life and death. Priority four do not get done. An example of priority four is for equipment that improves your quality of life. (Swain et al., 1998: 31)

Beattie et al. (2005) suggest that the underlying assumptions associated with the development of such instruments are that services are for people who cannot cope. In their research on dementia care services, they found that both family carers and GPs refrained from requesting services until they felt that the situation had become risky or dangerous.

The bureaucratization of social work and the growth of new managerialism have eroded the sphere of influence of the social work professional. Terms such as 'professional power' are probably too general and need to be deconstructed. Individual, front line social workers actually have very little power and influence over policy development, or in defining how resources are distributed.

What needs to change?

One way of mishandling change is to direct change at the wrong level of context. In this section of the chapter I will reflect upon what the possibilities of change are at the levels of the individual social worker, the organization and the policy context.

At the level of individual social work practice, social workers can:

- support disabled people to participate and define their own needs;
- share what power they have by sharing expertise and knowledge about the system and sources of support. This might include information about rights to independent advocates and procedures to appeal against decisions;
- encourage the active participation of disabled people in report writing or writing in case files. In this way, the voices of disabled people will be heard and represented in official documents and files;

- look for opportunities to work in partnership with disabled people – this will provide support to the practitioner as well as the disabled person;
- adopt the following guidelines when embarking on assessment with disabled people: clarify the goals towards which the person aspires; identify the barriers that may prevent the realization of these goals; work towards removing these barriers;
- privilege the disabled person's expertise (about their 'impairment' and the disabling barriers encountered) over professional expertise and theories;
- use concepts of reflective and reflexive practice to maintain ethical social work practice;
- adhere to social work values of inclusive working and valuing diversity.

At the level of organization social workers can:

- challenge unethical and discriminatory assessment tools and instruments;
- promote the development of inclusive practices and service user involvement in policy development;
- form alliances with other like-minded practitioners to promote change – there is safety in numbers!
- remember that they are professionals and use their professional power to influence orgainizational change;
- seek alliances and partnerships with disabled people's organizations.

At the level of policy social workers can:

- develop and maintain a political awareness of how government shapes major structures in society such as welfare and benefit policies;
- get involved! Remember and be proud of the radical and social reform traditions of the social work profession.

Conclusion

It could be argued that calling on individual social work practitioners to change policy or relinquish professional power is applying pressure for change at the wrong level of context. It may only result in disillusioned and deskilled practitioners consumed with guilt about not being able to change the 'system'. A better way may be to identify realizable change for practitioners that they can achieve in partnership with disabled people and with other like-minded colleagues. Success at this level may enable what is currently a disillusioned and often bullied workforce to push for change at other levels of the context, and to resurrect the notions of radicalism, collective action and social reform which were so central to the profession of social work in the past.

17 In Practice from the Viewpoint of Disabled People

Clare Evans

Faced with the harmful effects of professional policy, practice and provision what can disabled people themselves do to empower themselves and influence the services they receive? In the last twenty years, the Disabled People's Movement and the Independent Living Movement have organized themselves to challenge and influence professional social care provision and build a philosophy and services to support their concept of Independent Living. This chapter describes a model that has been used in two different contexts. It uses two main strategies to challenge professional policy, provision and practice from within a structure disabled people have created. The two strategies are supporting disabled people to empower themselves; and gaining power from professionals. One organization, Wiltshire and Swindon Users' Network, was formed by disabled people to challenge the local authority social care agenda and has been in existence for thirteen years; the other is the Leonard Cheshire Service Users Network Association (SUNA) and the Service Users Support Team (SUST) (together formally the Disabled People's Forum), which has developed over nine years. After this length of time it is possible to begin to assess what effect disabled people can have in isolating themselves from the harmful effects of professional intervention while being enabled to gain from the benefits of Independent Living as defined by disabled people.

The creation of dependency is an important issue to recognize when disabled people support others to organize and develop their own collective identity. Internalized dependency can make it difficult to reach many and mobilize them

(Continued)

(Continued)

to face challenges so it is necessary to develop an organizational culture built on disability quality principles and Independent Living. In Wiltshire, the new opportunities provided by the Community Care legislation to hear the voice of those who use services provided the initial impetus to self-organize, and this policy initiative gave professionals a reason to respond proactively. Substantial core funding, enabling the employment of disabled staff, provided from the 1993 community care infrastructure funding gave a firm base on which to develop an alternative cultural and structural framework based on disabled people's needs and valuing their expertise gained from experience. An invitation, a year later, to lead the development of a third-party scheme to provide cash payments to disabled people to purchase their own care enabled the principles of Independent Living to be fully explored and built into the organization.

The Leonard Cheshire organisations had been specialists in the provision of residential care for physically impaired disabled people for fifty years when in 1997 a successful bid for Lottery funding for the provision of training for service users provided the opportunity for disabled people to have sufficient resources to develop their own collective identity. It was then possible to apply a similar model to that used in Wiltshire and use disability equality and Independent Living training as a first tool to develop a wider network of service users. Leading trainers from the Independent Living movement were contracted to design and deliver 48-hour 'Disability Equality and Independent Living' courses at accessible hotels across the UK. For the first time for many disabled people, it was an opportunity to experience high levels of customer care and raise their aspirations beyond the institutions in which they lived. For others living in the community, the experience of sharing such thinking with other disabled people gave them their first opportunity to experience through empowerment the collective voice. From these courses it was a small step to show the need for ongoing development work to enable course participants and other disabled people who used Leonard Cheshire services to meet regularly to develop their own agenda and seek to challenge their service provider, Leonard Cheshire.

Principles of self-organization

The development of the collective organization in both contexts was led by clear principles that countered the prevailing professional values and stressed the importance of user expertise in all policy and service planning and development. The collective was organized on democratic principles and stressed the importance of 'hard to reach' service users, for example those with communication impairments. It recognized the need to fund the costs of disabled people meeting by reimbursing travel and care support costs. In Wiltshire it was an important principle of negotiating local authority funding also to pay an hourly rate to service users for working with professionals, all of whom were themselves paid to attend the meeting. Within Leonard Cheshire, the personal circumstance and rules of the Benefits Agency, together with the high costs of national travel and support costs, led disabled people to decide that reimbursement of expenses was their particular choice for recognition of their contribution.

Any organization disabled people establish to meet their needs must recognize the full meaning of empowerment (i.e. gaining control over one's life and having the ability to influence others) and its holistic implications for their lives. In Wiltshire, for example, during participation in the early training for care managers, assessments began with two questions: what kind of life do you want to lead? and what support do you want in order to achieve it? In Leonard Cheshire it has been possible to take this principle further due to the award in 2000 of further Lottery funding to employ disabled people as mentors. Their role is to work on a one-to-one basis with individual service users to assist them in identifying their aspirations and enable them to plan how to achieve these step by step. For some, this has meant what may appear as seemingly small steps to outsiders but to the individual is a very concrete achievement, such as leaving their room to use the computer room, while others have been able to use mentoring to move towards Independent Living or a community activity such as attending college. Throughout this mentoring the control remains with the service user, and that is a new experience for many of them.

The role of allies

Disabled people's organizations need to recognize the informal and formal power relations within which they work. Whilst being near the bottom of the formal power structure, disabled people have experienced a growth in informal power as the organization increased its influence. Key to this has been the role of allies in senior management positions within social care. Allies can share power and support disabled people in two ways: by leading from the front in valuing disabled people's expertise and recognizing their right to organize through key messages they send out; and by building personal links with the leaders of the disabled people's collective. In Wiltshire, the Director of Social Service's personal commitment and understanding influenced his managers and meant that the users' voice both individually and collectively took precedence. Consequently a gradual culture change took place so that managers at different levels became proactive in approaching the users' network for user involvement in any development of services.

The effect of this culture change on the pattern of service and the relationship with care managers was noticeable when comparing experiences with disabled people from other authorities. Financial resources to organize and run the user led organization were also protected by this key ally despite changes in the wider context, such as pressures from compulsory competitive tendering legislation from the European Community and Best Value Reviews affecting most funding applications. Initially, the service-level agreement only specified broad areas of work in exchange for funding, which gave flexibility for service users to set the agenda. But in the later, changed context, the Director negotiated a joint review process in recognition of the development work required to build such an organization and the inappropriateness of tendering for an external provider. However, too much reliance on individual allies and the lack of structural recognition of the need for ongoing service user involvement can lead to negative changes when the ally leaves his or her post. Indeed, this can threaten the funding of the organization itself, because the formal power structure has remained the same and the professionals retain the power to withdraw their support at any time. The Wiltshire and Swindon disabled people's organization still has its informal power and campaigning ability to challenge those decisions.

In Leonard Cheshire too, the support of senior managers in sending messages about the priority of valuing users' contributions and building personal links directly with disabled people gave an impetus to the development of user involvement. As Leonard Cheshire changed in response to the social policy context, the importance of service users' involvement as a matter of course became more widely recognized. Developing this model within a large voluntary organization, with the disabled manager reporting to the Director of Operations internally, brought the strength of gaining an understanding and personal knowledge of members of staff and structures within the organization whilst having the limitation of fears of possible repercussions from disabled people's challenges. This was partly offset by a recognition of the right of service users to challenge and receive support from disabled staff within the service users' support team. An independent evaluation by Professor John Swain and his team at Northumbria University identified patchy patterns of user involvement within the organization. In a subsequent action plan, developed from this evaluation, the need for corporate guidelines and the requirement of good practice in user involvement were identified. An accompanying User's Charter of expectations and rights is planned, to build the influence of disabled people into the structural power base of the organization.

Changing professional policy, provision and practice

How much can service users who have their own organizations and resources influence professional policy, practice and provision? Carr (2004), who carries out national research, found that service users feel they change practices very little as a result of their involvement. Certainly, to take on and try to change large bureaucracies which are part of the status quo needs enormous energy and application over time. Disabled people giving their views on one occasion can have little effect on established professional practice. This is reinforced by the way that professionals have been able to hijack the user involvement agenda. Since it has become good social policy practice to seek service users' views, some professionals have felt that to enable users to be involved and feel confident in doing so is in itself so empowering that the result of their involvement in relation to change is not important. In this context, only the ongoing strength of a user-controlled organisation able to develop its own agenda in some measure and to exert pressure over time can hope to create change in professional practice. In Wiltshire we worked to a policy of 'riddling the system' with users' perspectives at all stages of development practice and evaluation, hoping to bring about a change in the culture of the local authority social service department in addition to any one-off changes we desired. Following the disabled people's movement's catchphrase, 'Nothing about us, without us', we demanded to be involved at the start of every development in service. Certainly four years on, the Director of Social Services recognized, at a public meeting, that he felt 'thoroughly riddled'! Without a systematic evaluation from the start it is impossible to be sure how much of the culture change within the department was caused by service users pressing for change from the bottom up rather than by top-down central government messages about the importance of user involvement.

There were also particular achievements, such as service users influencing the development of care management procedures, paperwork built on the social model of disability, and influencing elected members to amend proposals being brought to Committee in such a way as to assist service users. All levels of the organization had direct service user involvement in different forms, from the prioritizing of standards for the Home Care Service to regular contact with elected members. The latter developed after a joint initiative between the Director of Social Services and the users' network to consult on the design of the kind of involvement users sought with elected members. Service users identified that it was potentially more powerful to influence members before they went into the council chamber and their views on policy were set along political party lines. Regular briefing meetings between the leading social care councillors and elected representatives from the users' network were consequently set up. Although at first these meetings were based on the committee agenda papers, service users soon negotiated an extension of the meeting to include their own agenda items too.

In Leonard Cheshire it has been harder to establish a comprehensive system of user involvement because of the widespread nature of the national organization's services and there were variations in how much we could do to influence services and challenge the resistance of some managers. Most service users decided that the changes they most sought were at service delivery level, in order to improve their everyday experience. Seeking to empower residential service users, traditionally identified as a hard to reach group, needed considerable amounts of facilitation and training before service provision could be influenced. Thus disabled staff employed as facilitators gathered service users together regularly to support them in identifying issues to influence and then to assist them by arranging training to enable them to be effective at lobbying. Some disabled people were happy to go forward to first of all design the process and then to participate in the national Committee of Service Users, whose chair became a trustee. Through this, it was possible to bring about changes which affected all service users. For example, it was the users' committee's pressure on directors that enabled residents to have access to at least one computer with internet access for their own use within each establishment.

So often changes in service users' experience of provision can require a change of staff, if service users identify that the process of including staff attitude and shortage of staff in the service delivery cannot be separated from the outcome of the service. User involvement in staff recruitment and selection is therefore important at all levels of Leonard Cheshire. Disabled staff in the Service Users' Support Team design and deliver training to service users to enable them to develop the skills needed to participate effectively in the recruitment process. A recent new development has been the involvement of members of the National Committee of SUNA on the panel selecting new trustees. It is hoped that plans to develop a Users' Charter and accompanying formal guidelines on user involvement, to be adopted by directors and endorsed by trustees, will lead to more consistent influence by service users within Leonard Cheshire.

Evaluating quality

The national policy emphasis on the outcomes for service users of professional practice and provision provides new opportunities for service users to be involved and give views that can lead to change. However, consumerist patterns of collecting users' views, such as paper questionnaires, will have limited use in this because of the low expectations created in some disabled people by the dependency-encouraging attitudes of professionals. The effects of this can be remedied somewhat if service users are involved in the design of the surveys in order to ensure that the priorities that users want to see within their service provision are the ones professionals measure in the survey. Whilst no disabled person can speak with complete knowledge of another service user's experience, it is noticeable how many of their views coincide and, though questionnaire surveys will always have a limited value, these users' priorities are often similar. A range of ways of collecting disabled people's views on services must be used in order for the quality of service to be designed by disabled people. Often more importantly, disabled people need to be involved in the design of questionnaires and other research tools.

In Wiltshire, the opportunity for disabled people to carry out a user-controlled best value review of direct payments demonstrated the value of users defining quality of service (Evans and Carmichael, 2002). Disabled people in the project group were able to develop a range of opportunities to collect all Direct Payment users' views. They decided to prioritize the quality of the Direct Payments Support Service and the local authority administrative requirements as issues needing addressing. At a time when Best Value Review processes were still developing, and with the Director of Social Services as an ally in identifying the role of 'user-controlled research', it was possible with the resources provided by the Joseph Rowntree Foundation to make this project a national demonstrative example of user-controlled service user involvement.

In Leonard Cheshire, also, service users have become increasingly involved in the quality agenda by the internal service audit process of the organisation. A team of service users, selected for their strength in this area from volunteers, have been trained to be regular members of the audit teams which visit each service to report once in four years. They are treated as full and equal members of the audit team and have particular strengths in interviewing service users. All service users are assisted in the audit by the SUST's facilitators and mentors, independent of the service provider staff, to reflect and prepare their views of the service ready to give to the audit team. Building this provision into the formal processes of the audit review enables all service users to feed into the process.

Conclusion

A professional once commented, 'We spend so much time considering how to support service users to empower themselves but it would be better if we could stop them being disempowered in the first place' (personal communication). This remains the challenge for professionals in examining and changing their policy practice and provision. Meanwhile, disabled people can seize the opportunity both to influence their practice and to build their own concepts of independent living and disability equality by joining together to develop a collective voice. If this voice is to be fully inclusive of marginalized service users, such organizations must have sufficient resources to develop a sound infrastructure so that they can reach out to all service users and challenge professional practice. The current social policy rhetoric of user-led outcomes is at odds with the realities of decreased funding to local disabled people's organizations and to social care provision funding. If the message of the Department of Health 2005 Green Paper is to be realized, disabled people need their own strong organizations to support them with information provision, training and peer support if they are to avoid the effects of dependency and disempowerment created by previous generations of professionals.

Conclusion: Some Reflections on Key Questions

In planning, compiling and editing this book we set out to explore and examine disability issues from a particular position: an affirmative, non-tragic model of disability and impairment. In doing so, however, we wished to document the complexities as well as the multifaceted and challenging nature of such a position. Drawing conclusions is a difficult task without diminishing the discussions and analyses presented in these chapters. Crucial has been the questioning of presumptions about the meaning of disability and impairment in peoples' lives.

To assist you as a reader of the text we provided Key Questions to Address in the introductory chapters to each section. It is not the purpose of this concluding chapter to attempt to provide 'the' answers to the questions we set. The purpose of the exercises has been to promote critical thinking and discussion. We hope that, like us, you found the ideas simulating, thought-provoking and challenging, at times reaffirming and at times contradicting your own thinking.

The chapters in Section I delved into manifestations and expressions of the tragedy model of disability and impairment. This is founded in beliefs that equate disabled people with suffering, abnormality, dependency, lack and loss, and the impossibility of valuing the self and leading valued lifestyles. Disabled people can find themselves 'prisoners of the misconceptions of others' (Gray and Hahn, 1997: 395), though, as is clear in the chapters in Section II, prisoners capable of resilience and resistance. The tragedy model, however, goes well beyond negative attitudes, beliefs or ways of thinking into inhumanity and personal and institutionalised abuse, as is graphically documented in Section I.

Perhaps the most difficult questions to address relate to why this is the dominant understanding of disability. Why the continuing inhuman treatment of disabled people? Is inhumanity built into our very nature as human beings? Section I invited you to explore the roots of the oppression of people with impairments, beliefs that are created and constructed within and by society.

Section II invited you to reflect on a affirmative, non-tragedy view of disability and impairment. We hope you found the Key Questions to Address complex, challenging and, as with the tragedy model, deeply rooted in what we are as human beings, individually and collectively. It is perhaps easier to say what an affirmative model is not about. First, it is not about all people with impairments celebrating difference. It is not about disabled people 'coming to terms with' disability and impairment. It is also not about disabled people being 'can do' or 'lovely' people. Finally, it is certainly not about the benefits of living and being marginalized and segregated within a disablist society.

As demonstrated in these chapters, affirmation is about being different and thinking differently about being different. The affirmative model is about disabled people challenging presumptions about themselves and their lives in terms of not only how they differ from what is average or normal, but also about the assertion, on disabled people's terms, of human embodiment, lifestyles, quality of life and identity. As the chapters in this section illustrate this is expressed both individually and collectively. Impairment is a part of human diversity, a phenomenon integral to the human condition, and reveals a significant understanding of humanity. There is also an affirmation of unique ways of being situated in society. As stated above, this is not an affirmation of disablement and there is a danger that it could be misinterpreted as 'a good life' in the face of oppression or segregation. However, disabled people can and do affirm ways of being and living that embrace difference. Take, for instance, parenting. A disabled father stated: 'I'm happy just to let them do things at their own pace, however slow that may be. It suits children to move slowly because it's more their pace' (Wates, 1997: 49). Wates takes this into the collective: 'disabled parents are able to offer their children and their children's friends something unique; the opportunity to learn about the meaning of disability in the context of close human relationships, rather than through the mesh of society's ignorance and prejudice' (1997: 46). 'Nothing about us without us' has been a key slogan of the disabled people's movement. By implication, the analyses within the chapters in this section augment this demand: 'on our terms'.

The chapters in Section III turned to possible implications of alternative ways of thinking within professional policy, provision of services and practice. The central proposition of this book can be stated as follows:

> Once an affirmative model of disability is accepted the goals of striving for physical independence and 'normality' become far less tenable. If disability is viewed as 'out there' in the environment and if disabled people are comfortable with themselves as they are, where does that leave providers of health and social care?

As is apparent in the Key Questions to Address, there are numerous issues. There are no clearly defined formulas for change here. There is no comfortable remit. The affirmative model itself does not provide a different set of presumptions to replace those that characterize individual models, particularly the tragedy model. It is as ludicrous to presume that a disabled person is comfortable with him/herself as he/she is as to presume that his/her life is devastated by impairment. Equally, implications of the affirmative model challenge traditional approaches to health and social care, prioritizing cure or care, and the worst manifestations can be conceived of and experienced as abuse – 'care' as abuse. Yet this does not negate the potential usefulness to disabled people of the skills of service providers or the need for support.

For us the realization of 'disability on equal terms' lies in principles that are underpinned by an affirmative model. We would tentatively suggest the following.

- confronting personal and institutionalized presumptions about the meaning of impairment and disability and about the lives and aspirations of disabled people;
- moving away from a client-based approach in service provision towards a citizen-based model where service users are fully involved in the formulation and running of services themselves at all stages, including the production of knowledge about what disability is and what services, if any, are required;
- questioning professional agendas for change coming under such 'new initiatives' as multi-professional practice, empowerment and partnership, particularly in terms of the views and experiences of those on the receiving end – service users;
- understanding and valuing difference in health and social care that is truly inclusive for all: working towards full participative citizenship irrespective of age, gender, ethnicity, sexuality – and disability and impairment.

References

Abberley, P. (1995) 'Disabling ideology in health and welfare – The case of occupational therapy', *Disability and Society*, 10: 221–232.

Abbott, P. and Meerabaeu, L. (eds) (1998) *The Sociology of the Caring Professions*. London: University College London Press.

Abelow Hedley, L. (2006) 'The seduction of the surgical fix', in E. Parens (ed.) *Surgically Shaping Children: Technology, Ethics and the Pursuit of Normality*. Baltimore: Johns Hopkins University Press.

Abercrombie, N. (1996) *Television and Society*. Cambridge: Polity Press.

Ablon, J. (1990) 'Ambiguity and difference: families with dwarf children', *Social Science and Medicine*, 30(8): 879–887.

Agle, D. (1964) 'Psychiatric studies of patients with haemophilia and related states', *Archives of Internal Medicine*, 114: 76–82.

Allen, J. (2005) 'Encounters with exclusion through disability arts', *Journal of Research in Special Educational Needs*, 5(1): 31–36.

Anjali website: www.anjali.co.uk (visited 25 July 2006).

Arnstein, S.R. (1969) 'A ladder of citizen participation', *Journal of the American Institute of Planners*, 35(4): 216–224.

Asch, A. (2001) 'Disability, bioethics and human rights', in G. Albrecht, K.D. Seelman and M. Bury (eds) *Handbook of Disability Studies*. London: Sage.

Aspinall, C. (2006) 'Do I make you uncomfortable? Reflecting on using surgery to reduce the distress of others', in E. Parens (ed.) *Surgically Shaping Children: Technology, Ethics and the Pursuit of Technology*. Baltimore: Johns Hopkins University Press.

Aznar, J., Magallon, M., Querol, F., Gorina, E. & Tusell, J. (2000) The orthopaedic status of severe haemophiliacs in Spain. *Haemophilia*, 6: 170–176.

Bailey, R. and Brake, M. (1975) *Radical Social Work Practice*. London: Arnold.

Baker, M. (1990) *Who All Hopes Dashed in the Human Zoo*. Warminster: Danny Howell Books.

Band, R. (1997) *Getting Better. How People with Learning Disabilities Can Get the Best from their GP.* Brighton: Pavilion Publishing.

Banks, S. and Williams R. (2005) 'Accounting for ethical difficulties in social welfare work: issues, problems and dilemmas', *British Journal of Social Work*, 35: 1005–1022.

Barber, R. in Wright, C. and Rowe, N. (2005) Protecting Professional Identities: Service User Involvement and Occupational Therapy, *British Journal of Occupational Therapy*, 68(1): 45–47

Barnes, C. (1994) 'Images of disability', in S. French (ed.) *On Equal Terms: working with disabled people*. Oxford: Buttterworth-Heinemann.

Barnes, C. and Mercer, G. (eds) (1997) *Doing Disability Research*. Leeds: The Disability Press.

Barnes, C. and Mercer, G. (2003) *Disability*. Cambridge: Polity Press.

Barnes, C. and Mercer, G. (2005) *The Social Model of Disability: Europe and the majority world*. Leeds: The Disability Press.

Barnes C. and Mercer G. (2006) *Independent Futures: creating user-led disability services in a disabling society*. Bristol: Policy Press.

Barnes, C. and Roulstone, A. (2005) '"Work" is a four-letter word: disability, work and welfare', in A. Roulstone and C. Barnes (eds) *Working Futures? Disabled people, policy and social inclusion*.

Barnes, C., Mercer, G. and Shakespeare, T. (1999) *Exploring Disability: a sociological introduction*. Cambridge: Polity Press.

Baum, C. and Christianson, C. (1997) 'The occupational therapy context', in C. Christianson and C. Baum (eds) *Occupational Therapy: Enabling Function and Well Being*, 2nd edn. Slack: Thorafare.

BBC 3 broadcast 6 April 2006 'I love being mad'. Available online: http://www.bbc.co.uk/bbc three/tv/ilove_mad.shtml (visited 1 October 2006).

Beattie, A., Daker-White, G., Gilliard, J. and Means, R. (2005) '"They don't quite fit the way we organise our services" – results from a UK field study of marginalised groups and dementia care', *Disability and Society*, 20(1): 47–80.

Beresford, P. (2000) 'What have madness and psychiatric systems survivors got to do with disability and disability studies?' *Disability and Society*, 15(1): 167–172.

Beresford, P. and Croft, S. (1986) *Whose Welfare: Private Care or Public Services?* Brighton: Lewis Cohen Urban Studies Centre.

Beresford, P. and Croft, S. (2000) 'User involvement', in M. Davies (ed.) *The Blackwell Encyclopaedia of Social Work*. Oxford: Blackwell.

Beresford, P., Croft, S., Evans, C. and Harding, T. (1997) 'Quality in personal social services: the developing role of user involvement in the UK', in A. Evans, K. Haverinan, K. Leichsering and G. Wistow (eds) *Developing Quality in Personal Social Services*. Aldershot: Ashgate.

Beresford, P., Croft, S., Evans, C. and Harding, T. (2000) 'Quality in personal social services: the developing role of user involvement in the UK', in C. Davies, L. Finlay and A. Bullman (eds) *Changing Practice in Health and Social Care*. London: Sage.

Berger, P. and Luckmann, T. (1984) *The Social Construction of Reality: a treatise on the sociology of knowledge*. Harmondsworth: Penguin.

Bogdan, R. (1996) 'The social construction of freaks', in R. Garland Thomson (ed.) *Freakery: Cultural Spectacles of the Ordinary Body*. New York: New York University Press.

Bogdan, R. and Taylor, S. (1976) 'The judged, not the judges: an insider's view of mental retardation', *American Psychologist*, 31(1): 47–52.

Bolen, R. (2002) 'Child sexual abuse and attachment theory: are we rushing headlong into another controversy?' *Journal of Child Sexual Abuse*, 11(1): 95–124.

Booth, T. and Booth, W. (1997) 'Making connections: a narrative study of adult children of parents with learning difficulties', in C. Barnes and G. Mercer (eds) *Doing Disability Research*. Leeds: The Disability Press.

Borsay, A. (2005) *Disability and Social Policy in Britain since 1750: a history of exclusion*. Basingstoke: Palgrave Macmillan.

Brandon, D. (1981) *Voices of Experience: consumer perspectives of psychiatric treatment*. London: MIND.

Brandon, D. (1990) *Strange Places: experiences in a mental handicap hospital.* Salford: University College Salford.

Brandon, D. (1994) *Anglia Poems.* Cambridge: Anglia Polytechnic University.

Brandon, T. (2005) 'Empowerment, policy levels and service forums', *Journal of Learning Disabilities,* 9(4): 321–331.

Bridging the Gap: a guide to disabled student allowances (DSAs) in Higher Education 2005/2006. London: Department of Education and Skills.

Brisenden, S. (*c.*1987) *Poems for Perfect People* (Self-published, n.d.).

Buchanan, A., Brock, D.W., Daniels, N. and Wikler, D. (2000) *From Chance to Choice: genetics and justice.* Cambridge: Cambridge University Press.

Bullinger, M., Von Mackensen, S., Fischer, K., Khair, K., Petersen, C., Ravens-Sieberer, U., Rocino, A., Sagnier, P., Tusell, J., Van Den Berg, H. & Vicarot, M. (2002) 'Pilot testing of the 'Haemo-QoL' quality of life questionnaire for haemophiliac children in six European countries', *Haemophilia,* 8: 47–54.

Burchinall, P. (1982) 'Mental handicap nursing', in P. Allen, and M. Jolley (eds) *Nursing, Midwifery & Health Visiting since 1900.* London: Faber and Faber.

Bury, M. (1982) 'Chronic illness as biographical disruption', *Sociology of Health and Illness,* 4: 67–81.

Byng, S. & Duchan, J. (2005) 'Social model philosophies and principles: their applications to therapies for aphasia', *Aphasiology,* 19: 906–922.

Campbell, B. (1988) *Unofficial Secrets: child sexual Abuse – the Cleveland case.* London: Virago Press.

Campbell, J. and Oliver, M. (1996) *Disability Politics: understanding our past, changing our future.* London: Routledge.

Can't Do Nursing with One Hand: Nikki Heazell proves everyone wrong (2003), Open 4 All Campaign Material, London, Disability Rights Commission.

Caplan, A., McGee, G. and Magnus, D. (1999) 'What is immoral about eugenics?', *British Medical Journal,* 319: 441–444.

Carmichael, A. (2004) 'The social model, the emancipatory paradigm and user involvement', in C. Barnes and G. Mercer (eds) *Implementing the Social Model of Disability: theory and research.* Leeds: The Disability Press.

Carr, S. (2004) *Has Service User Involvement Made a Difference to Social Care Services?* London: Social Care Institute for Excellence.

Carter, S. (2000) 'Adding life to years as well as years to life: primary health care for people with learning difficulties', in R. Astor and K. Jeffries (eds) *Positive Initiatives for People with Learning Difficulties: promoting healthy lifestyles.* Basingstoke: Macmillan.

Carver, C. & Scheier, M. (2000) Scaling back goals and recalibration of the affect system are processes in normal adaptive self-regulation: understanding 'response shift' phenomena. *Social Science and Medicine,* 50: 1715–1722.

Casling, D. (1994) 'Art for whose sake?' *Disability and Society,* 9(3): 383–394.

Castor-Lewis, C. (1988) 'On doing research with adult incest survivors: some initial thoughts and considerations', *Women and Therapy,* 7(1): 73–80.

Cella, D. & Tulsky, D. (1990) 'Measuring quality of life today: methodological aspects', *Oncology,* May, 29–38.

Charlton, J. I. (1998). *Nothing About Us Without Us: disability oppression and empowerment.* California: University of California Press.

Childs, D.J. (2001) *Modernism and Eugenics : Woolf, Eliot, Yeats, and the culture of degeneration*. Cambridge: Cambridge University Press.

Choppin, E. (2006) 'Outcry over proposed killing of disabled babies', *Disability Now*, December.

Clare, J. (1997) *John Clare*. London: Orion.

Clarke, A. (1991) 'Is non-directive genetic counselling possible?' *The Lancet*, 338: 998–1000.

Coleridge, P. (1993) *Disability, Liberation and Development*. Oxford: Oxfam.

Collins J. (1992) *When the Eagles Fly: a report on the resettlement of people with learning difficulties from long-stay institutions*. London: Values Into Action.

Coombs R. (2004), April, *NHS Magazine Primary Care*, Department of Health.

Corker, M. (1996) *Deaf Transitions: images and origins of deaf families, deaf communities and deaf identities*. London: Jessica Kingsley.

Corker, M. and Shakespeare, T. (2002) *Disability/postmodernity: embodying disability theory*. London: Continuum.

COT (2002) *From Interface to Integration – A Strategy for Modernising Occupational Therapy Services in Local Health and Social Care Communities*. London: College of Occupational Therapists.

Craddock, J. (1996) 'Responses of the occupational therapy profession to the perspective of the disability movement', Part 2, *British Journal of Occupational Therapy*, 59(2): 73–78.

Creek, J. (2003) *Occupational Therapy Defined as a Complex Intervention*. London: College of Occupational Therapy.

Croft, S. and Beresford, P. (1989) 'User involvement, citizenship and social policy', *Critical Social Policy*, 26: 5–18.

Croft, S. and Beresford, P. (2002) 'Service users' perspectives', in M. Davies (ed.) *Companion to Social Work*, 2nd edn. Oxford: Blackwell.

Cumberbatch, G. and Negrine, R. (1992) *Images of Disability on Television*. London: Routledge.

Darke, P. (2004) 'The changing face of representation of disability in the media', in J. Swain, S. French, C. Barnes and C. Thomas (eds) *Disabling Barriers–Enabling Environments*, 2nd edn. London: Sage.

Davies, B.P. and Knapp, M.R.J. (1981) *Old People's Homes and the Production of Welfare*. London: Routledge, Kegan and Paul.

Davies, C. (1995) *Gender and the Professional Predicament*. Buckingham: Open University Press.

Davies, C. and Pointon, A. (1997) *Framed: interrogating disability in the media*. London: British Film Institute.

Davies, K. (1993) 'The crafting of good clients', in J. Swain, V. Finkelstein, S. French and M. Oliver (eds) *Disabling Barrier – Enabling Environments*. London: Sage.

Davis, K. (2004) 'The crafting of good clients', in J. Swain, S. French, C. Barnes and C. Thomas (eds) *Disabling Barriers – Enabling Environments*, 2nd edn. London: Sage.

Davis, J. and Watson, N. (2001) 'Where are the children's experiences? Analysing social and cultural exclusion in "special" and "mainstream" schools', *Disability and Society*, 16(5): 671–687.

Davis, L. (ed.) (1997) *The Disability Studies Reader*. London: Routledge.

Department for Education and Skills (2005/2006) *A guide to financial support for higher education students in 2005/2006*, London: Department for Education and Skills.

Department of Health (1998) *The Healthy Way*. London: HMSO.

Department of Health (1999) *National Service Framework for Mental Health: modern standards and service models*. London: Department of Health.

Department of Health (2000) *Looking beyond labels: Widening the employment opportunities for disabled people in the new NHS*, London: Department of Health.

Department of Health (2001a) *The National Health Inequalities Targets*. London: Department of Health.

Department of Health (2001b) *Valuing People: a new strategy for learning disability for the 21st century*. London: HMSO.

Desmond, A. and Moore, J. (1991) *Darwin: the life of a tormented evolutionist*. New York: Warner Books.

DHSS (1971) *Better Services for the Mentally Handicapped*. London: HMSO.

Different Differences Disability Equality Teaching in Healthcare Education: a document for action, produced by Partners in Practice, the University of Bristol, the University of the West of England and the Peninsula Medical School, Plymouth and Exeter.

Dikitter, F. (1998) *Imperfect Conceptions: medical knowledge, birth defects and eugenics in China*. New York: Columbia University Press.

Dimmock, A.F. (1993) *Cruel Legacy: an introduction to the record of deaf people in history*. Edinburgh: Scottish Workshop Publications.

Dingwall, R., Rafferty, A.M. and Webster, C. (1992) *An Introduction to the Social History of Nursing*. London: Routledge.

Disability Discrimination (2006) *A-Z Advice Sheet*. London: Nursing and Midwifry Council.

Disability and Difference (2002) Programme 1. Audio CD 2. *K202 Care Welfare and Community*. Milton Keynes: Open University.

Disability Rights Commission (2003) *Can't do Nursing with one Hand! – Nikki Heazell Proves Everyone Wrong*. Disability Rights Commission. http://www.drc-gb.org/newsroom/news details.asp?id=244§ion=1

Disability Rights Commission (2005) *Equality Duty Codes of Practice*. London.

Disch, E. (2001) 'Research as clinical practice: creating a positive research experience for survivors of sexual abuse by professionals', *Sociological Practice: A Journal of Clinical and Applied Sociology*, 3(3): 15–24.

Djulbegovic, B., Goldsmith, G., Vaughn, D., Birkimer, J., Marasa, M., Joseph, G., Huang, A. & Hadley, T. (1996) 'Comparison of the quality of life between HIV-positive haemophilia patients and HIV-negative haemophilia patients', *Haemophilia*, 2: 166–172.

Dodd, K. and Brunker, J. (1998) *Feeling Poorly*. Brighton: Pavilion Publishing.

Dominelli, L. (1998) 'Anti-oppressive practice in context', in R. Adams, L. Dominelli and M. Payne (eds) *Social Work: Themes, Issues and Critical Debates*. London: Macmillan.

Dooher, J. and Byrt, R. (2003) *Empowerment and the Health Service User*, Vol. 2. Wiltshire: Mark Allen.

Dowse, L. and Frohmader, C. (2001) *Moving Forward: sterilisation and reproductive health of women and girls with disabilities*. Tasmania: Women with Disabilities Australia.

Drake, R. H. (1996) 'A critique of the role of traditional charities', in L. Barton (ed.) *Disability and Society: emerging issues and insights*. London: Longman.

Duchan, J. (1999) Reports written by speech-language pathologists: the role of agenda in constructing client competence, in D. Korvarsky, J. Duchan and M. Maxwell (eds) *Constructing (In)competence: Disabling evaluation in clinical and social interaction*. London: Erlbaum.

Duchan, J. (ed.) (2006) 'Communication access models and methods for promoting social inclusion', *Topics in Language Disorders*, 26: 3.

Durham, A. (2003) *Young Men Surviving Child Sexual Abuse: research stories and lessons for therapeutic practice*. Hoboken, NJ: John Wiley and Sons.

Duster, T. (1990) *Backdoor to Eugenics*. New York: Routledge.

Eagle, M. (2003) *Images of Disability Annual Report.* Available: www.disability.gov.uk

Edwards, E. (ed.) (1992) *Anthropology and Photography 1860–1920.* London: Yale University Press.

Elliott, D. and Briere, J. (1995) 'Posttraumatic stress associated with delayed recall of sexual abuse: a general population study', *Journal of Traumatic Stress,* 8(4): 629–647.

Elliott, J. (2005) 'Crossing the jungle in a wheelchair' http://news.bbc.co.uk/1/hi/health/4319920 (17 November 2005)

Ellis, H. (1927) *The Task of Social Hygiene.* London: Constable.

Emerson, E. (1992) 'What is normalisation?' in H. Brown and H. Smith (eds) *Normalisation: a reader for the nineties.* London: Routledge.

Emerson, E. and Hatton, C. (1994) *Moving Out: relocation from hospital to community.* London: HSO.

Esland, G. (1980) 'Professions and professionalism', in G. Esland and G. Salaman (eds) *The Politics of Work and Occupations.* Milton Keynes: The Open University Press.

Evans C., Carmichael A. and members of the Direct Payment Best Value Project Group of Wiltshire and Swindon Users' Network (2002) *Users' Best Value: a guide to user involvement good practice in Best Value Reviews.* York: Joseph Rowntree Foundation.

Evans, J. and Hall, S. (eds) (1999) *Visual Culture: the reader.* London: Sage.

Evans, S.E. (2004) *Forgotten Crimes: the holocaust and people with disabilities.* Chicago, IL: Ivan R. Dee.

Evans, W. and Maines, D. (1995) 'Narrative structures and the analysis of incest', *Symbolic Interaction,* 18(3): 303–322.

Ewing, W.A. (1994) *The Body: photoworks of the human form.* London: Thames and Hudson.

Fawcett, B. (2000) *Feminist Perspectives on Disability.* London: Prentice-Hall.

Ferguson, I. (2003) 'Challenging a "spoiled identity": mental health service users, recognition and redistribution', in S. Riddell and N. Watson (eds) *Disability, Culture and Identity.* Harlow: Pearson Education.

Fergusson, R., Hughes, G. and Neal, S. (2004) 'Welfare - from security to responsibility?' in G. Hughes and R. Fergusson (eds) *Ordering Lives: family, world and welfare,* 2nd edn. London: Routledge.

Finkelstein, V. (1980) *Attitudes and Disabled People: issues for discussion.* New York: Rehabilitation Fund.

Finkelstein, V. (1987) 'Disabled people and our cultural development', *DAIL,* 8, June.

Finkelstein, V. (2004) 'Modernising services?' in J. Swain, S. French, C. Barnes and C. Thomas (eds) *Disabling Barriers – Enabling Environments,* 2nd edn. London: Sage.

Finkelstein, V. and Morrison, E. (1993) *Broken Arts and Cultural Repair: the role of culture in the empowerment of disabled people.* In Swain, J. V. Finkelstein, S. French and M. Oliver (eds) *Disabling Barriers – Enabling Environments.* London: Sage.

Finkelstein, V., French, S. and Oliver, M. (eds) *Disabling Barriers – Enabling Environments.* London: Sage.

Firth, H. (1986) *A Move to Community: social contacts and behaviour.* Morpeth: Northumberland Health Authority.

Fischer, K., Van Der Bom, J. & Van Den Berg, H. (2003) Health-related quality of life as an outcome parameter in haemophilia treatment, *Haemophilia,* 9: 75–82.

Fleming, J., Mullen, P.E., Sibthorpe, B. and Bammer, G (1999) 'The long-term impact of childhood sexual abuse in Australian women', *Child Abuse and Neglect,* 23(2): 145–159.

Foucault, M. (1973) *The Birth of the Clinic: an archaeology of medical perception.* London: Tavistock.

Foucault, M. (1977) *Discipline and Punish: the birth of the prison.* London: Allen Lane.

Foucault, M. (1980) *Power and Knowledge.* Brighton: Harvester.

Frank, A.W. (1995) *The Wounded Storyteller: body, illness and ethics*. Chicago: University of Chicago Press.

Fraser, N. (2000) 'Rethinking recognition', *New Left Review*, 3: 107–120.

Freire, P. (1972) *Pedagogy of the Oppressed*. London: Sheen and Ward.

French, S. (1990) 'The advantages of visual impairment: some physiotherapists' views', *The New Beacon*, 74 (872): 1–6.

French, S. (ed.) (1994a) *On Equal Terms: working with disabled people*. Oxford: Butterworth-Heinemann.

French, S. (1994b) 'The disabled role', in S. French (ed.) *On Equal Terms: working with disabled people*. Oxford: Butterworth-Heinemann.

French, S. (1997) 'Inequalities in health', in S. French (ed.) *Physiotherapy: a psychosocial approach*, 2nd edn. Oxford: Butterworth-Heinemann.

French, S. (2004) '"Can you see the rainbow?" The roots of denial', in J. Swain, S. French, C. Barnes and C. Thomas (eds) *Disabling Barriers–Enabling Environments*, 2nd edn. London: Sage.

French, S. (2004) 'Enabling relationships in therapy practice', in J. Swain, J. Clark, S. French, F. Reynolds and K. Parry *Enabling Relationships in Health and social Care*. Oxford: Butterworth-Heinemann.

French, S. and Swain, J. (1998) 'Normality and disabling care', in A. Brechin, J. Walmsley, J. Katz and S. Peace (eds) *Care Matters: concepts, practice and research*. London: Sage.

French, S. and Swain, J. (2001) 'The relationship between disabled people and health and welfare professionals', in G. Albrecht, K.D. Seelman and M. Bury (eds) *Handbook of Disability Studies*. London: Sage.

French, S. and Swain, J. (2004) 'Whose tragedy? Towards a personal non-tragedy view of disability', in J. Swain, S. French, C. Barnes and C. Thomas (eds) *Disabling Barriers–Enabling Environments*, 2nd edn. London: Sage.

French, S. with Swain, J., Atkinson, D. and Moore, M. (2006) *An Oral History of the Education of Visually Impaired People: telling stories for inclusive futures*. Lampeter: The Edwin Mellen Press.

Friedson, E. (1994) *Professionalism Reborn: theory, prophecy and policy*. Cambridge: Polity Press.

Fromuth, M. E. (1986) 'The relationship of childhood sexual abuse with later psychological and sexual adjustment in a sample of college women', *Child Abuse and Neglect*, 10: 5–15.

Fry, S. (2006) 'The secret life of the manic depressive', BBC TV broadcast 19 September 2006. Available online: http://www.bbc.co.uk/bbctwo/programmes/?id=manic_depressive

Furgusson, R., Hughes, G. and Neal, S. (2004) 'Welfare: from security to responsibility?' in G. Hughes and R. Furgusson (eds) *Ordering Lives: family, work and welfare*, 2nd edn. London: Routledge.

Gaarder, E. (2000) 'Gender politics: the focus on women in the memory debates', *Journal of Child Sexual Abuse*, 9(1): 91–106.

Galipeault, J.P. (2003) as cited in Townsend, E. (2003) 'Reflections on power and justice in enabling occupation', *The Canadian Journal of Occupational Therapy*, 70(2): 74–157.

Galvin, R. (2003) 'The paradox of disability culture: the need to combine versus the imperative to let go', *Disability and Society*, 18(5): 675–690.

Gauntlett, D. and Hill, A. (1999) *TV Living: television, culture and everyday life*. London: Routledge.

General Social Care Council (2002) *New Requirements for the Award of the Social Work Degree*. London: General Social Care Council.

General Social Care Council (2004) *The Revised Post Qualifying Framework for Social Work Education and Training*. London: General Social Care Council.

Gibbs, D. (2004) 'Social model services: an oxymoron?' in C. Barnes and G. Mercer (eds) *Disability Policy And Practice: applying the social model.* Leeds: The Disability Press.

Giddens, A. (1991) *Modernity and Self Identity: self and society in the late modern age.* Cambridge: Polity Press.

Gilgun, J. and Reiser, E. (1990) 'The development of sexual identity among men sexually abused as children', *Families in Society: The Journal of Contemporary Human Services,* November 71: (9): 515–523.

Gillman, M., Swain, J. and Heyman, B. (1997) 'Life history or "case" history: the objectification of people with learning difficulties through the tyranny of professional discourses', *Disability & Society,* 12: 675–693.

Gleeson, B. (1999) *Geographies of Disability.* London: Routledge.

Glover, J. (1984) *What Sort of People Should There Be?* Harmondsworth: Penguin.

Glover, J. (1999) 'Eugenics and human rights', in J. Burley (ed.) *The Genetic Revolution and Human Rights.* Oxford: Oxford University Press.

Goble, C. (2000) 'Partnership in residential settings', in R. Astor and K. Jeffries (eds) *Positive Initiatives for People with Learning Difficulties: promoting healthy lifestyles.* Basingstoke: Macmillan.

Goble, C. (2004) 'Dependence, independence and normality', in J. Swain, S. French, C. Barnes and C. Thomas (eds) *Disabling Barriers – Enabling Environments,* 2nd edn. London: Sage.

Goffman, E. (1961) *Asylums.* Harmondsworth: Penguin.

Goffman, E. (1963) *Stigma: notes on the management of spoiled identity.* Englewood Cliffs, New Jersey: Prentice-Hall.

Gomm, R. (1993) 'Issues of power in health and welfare', in J. Walmsley, J. Reynolds, P. Shakespeare and R. Woolfe (eds) *Health, Welfare and Practice: reflecting on roles and relationships.* London: Sage.

Goren, H. (2002) 'Occupational therapy and strictly defined areas of doubt and uncertainty', *British Journal of Occupational Therapy,* 65(10): 476–478.

Gray, D.B. and Hahn, (1997) Achieving occupational goals: the social effects of stigma, in C. Christiansen and C. Baum (eds) *Occupational Therapy: Enabling function and well-being.* Thorofare, NJ: Slack.

Gray, B. and Ridden, G. (1999) *Lifemaps of People with Learning Disabilities.* London: Jessica Kingsley.

Greenhaulgh, L. (1994) *Well Aware: improving access to health information for people with learning difficulties.* Anglia and Oxford Regional Health Authority/NHS Executive.

Gregory, A. (2003) *Eureka! The birth of science.* London: Icon Books.

Gringeri, A., Mantovani, L., Scalone, L., Mannucci, P. & COCIS Study Group. (2003) 'Cost of care and quality of life for patients with hemophilia complicated by inhibitors: the COCIS study group' *Blood,* 102, 2358–2363.

Gross, R. (1995) *Psychology: the science of mind and behaviour.* Sevenoaks: Hodder and Stoughton.

Halifax, J. (1981) *Shaman the Wounded Healer.* London: Thames and Hudson.

Hammell, K.A. (1998) 'From the Neck Up: quality of life following high spinal cord injury'. Ph.D. thesis, University of British Columbia, Vancouver, Canada.

Hammel, K.W. (2004) 'Deviating from the norm: a sceptical interrogation of The Classifactory Practices of the ICF', *British Journal of Occupational Therapy,* 67(9): 408–411.

Hampton, S.J. (2005) 'Family eugenics', *Disability and Society,* 20(5): 553–561.

Handy, C. (1990) *The Age of Unreason.* London: Arrow.

Handy, C. (1999) *Understanding Organizations.* London: Penguin.

Harrison, R., Mann, G., Murphy, M., Taylor, A. and Thompson N. (2003) *Partnership Made Painless: a joined-up guide to working together*. London: Russell House.

Hart, S. (2003) 'Health and health promotion', in B. Gates (ed.) *Learning Disabilities: towards inclusion*. London: Churchill Livingstone.

Hays, R. & Shapiro, M. (1992) 'An overview of generic health-related quality of life measures for HIV research', *Quality of Life Research*, 1: 91–97.

Heart 'n Soul website: www.heartsoul.co.uk (visited 20 July 2006).

Heenan, D. (2006) 'Art as therapy: an effective way of promoting positive mental health?' *Disability and Society*, 21(2): 179–191.

Heenan, D. (1996) 'Art as therapy: an effective way of presenting positive mental health?', *Disability and Society*, 21(2): 179–191.

Heraud, B (1973) 'Professionalism, radicalism and social change', in P. Halmos (ed.) *Professionalisation and Social Change*. University of Keele Monograph, No 20. Keele: University of Keele.

Hernandez, J., Gray, D. & Lineberger, H. (1989) 'Social and economic indicators of well being among hemophiliacs over a 5-year period', *General Hospital Psychiatry*, 11: 241–247.

Hetherington, K. (1998) *Expressions of Identity: space, performance, politics*. London: Sage.

Hevey, D. (1992) *The Creatures Time Forgot: photography and disability imagery*. London: Routledge.

Hewerdine, F. and Laugesen, L. (2005) 'Victims? – not a bit of it', *Speech and Language Therapy in Practice*, Spring: 10–13

Hewitt, A. and Byng, C. (2003) 'From doing to being: from participation to engagement', in S. Parr, J. Duchan and C. Pound (eds) *Aphasia Inside Out*. Maidenhead: Open University Press.

Higgins, M. (2006) *An exploration of the lives of disabled people sexually abused in childhood: "the double whammy effect"*. Ph.D. thesis, Northumbria University.

Hilty, G. (2004) www.fourthplinth.co.uk/press_release, 16 June.

Holdsworth, A. (1988) Sleeve notes to *Choices and Rights* tape compilation. http://www.disabilityarts.com/chronology/

Holliday Willey, L. (1999) *Pretending to be Normal: living with Asperger's Syndrome*. London: Jessica Kingsley.

Hughes, G. and Lewis, G. (1996) *Unsettling Welfare: the reconstruction of social policy*. London: Routledge.

Hughes, B. (2002) 'Bauman's Strangers: impairment and the invalidation of disabled people in modern and post modern cultures', *Disability and Society*, 17(5): 571–584.

Hull and Holderness Community Health NHS Trust (1995) *The Patient's Charter and You, with Signs and Symbols*. Hull and Holderness NHS Trust and Makaton Vocabulary Development Project.

Humphries, S. and Gordon, P. (1992) *Out of Sight: the experience of disability 1900–1950*. Plymouth: Northcote House.

Humphreys, S., Evans, G. and Todd, S. (1987) *Lifelines: an account of the experiences of seven people with a mental handicap who use the nimrod service*. London: King's Fund.

Humphries, B. (2004) 'An unacceptable role for social work: implementing immigration policy', *British Journal of Social Work*, 34: 93–107.

Hunt, P. (1966) *Stigma: the experience of disability*. London: Chapman.

Huxley, A. (2004) *The Doors of Perception, and Heaven and Hell*. London: Vintage.

Ingstad, B. and Reynolds Whyte, S. (eds) (1995) *Disability and Culture*. Los Angeles: University of California Press.

Ireland, C. (1999). *Creative Window Truthteller*. Unpublished.

Jackson, M. (1996) 'Institutional provision for the feeble-minded in Edwardian England: Sandlebridge and the scientific morality of permanent care', in D. Wright and A. Digby (eds) *From Idiocy to Mental Deficiency: historical perspectives on people with learning disabilities*. London: Routledge.

Jamison, K. R. (1993) *Touched with Fire*. London: Free Press.

Jenkins, R. (1996) *Social Identity*. London: Routledge.

Johnson, K. and Traustadottir, R. (2005) *Deinstitutionalisation and People with Intellectual Disabilities: in and out of institutions*. London: Jessica Kingsley.

Jones, C., Ferguson, I., Lavalette, M. and Penketh, L. (2006) *Social work and social justice: a manifesto for a new engaged practice*. www.liv.ac.uk/ssp/Social_Work_Manifesto.html

Kagan, A. (1998) 'Supported conversation for adults with aphasia: methods and resources for training conversation partners', *Aphasiology*, 12: 816–830.

Keith, L. (2001) *Take Up Thy Bed and Walk: death, disability and cure in classic fiction for girls*. London: The Women's Press.

Kelves, D. (1995) *In the Name of Eugenics: genetics and the uses of human heredity*. Cambridge, MA: Harvard University Press.

Kenny, K. (2001) 'Child abuse reporting: teachers' perceived deterrents', *Child Abuse and Neglect*, 25: 81–92.

Kent, D. (2000) 'Somewhere a mocking bird', in E. Parens and A. Asch (eds) *Prenatal Testing and Disability Rights*. Washington, DC: Georgetown University Press.

Kerr, A. and Shakespeare, T. (2002) *Genetic Politics: from eugenics to genome*. Cheltenham: New Clarion Press.

Kerr, A., Cunningham-Burley, S. and Amos, A. (1998) 'Eugenics and the new human genetics in Britain: examining contemporary professionals', accounts', *Science, Technology and Human Values*, 23(2): 175–198.

Kevles, D.J. (1985) *In the Name of Eugenics: genetics and the uses of human heredity*. New York: Knopf.

Khosa, J. (2003) 'Still Life of a Chameleon: aphasia and its impact on identity', in S. Parr, J. Duchan and C. Pound (eds) *Aphasia Inside Out*. Maidenhead: Open University Press.

Kielhofner, G. (2005) 'Rethinking disability and what to do about it: disability studies and its implications for occupational therapy', *The American Journal of Occupational Therapy*, 59(5): 487–496.

Kitcher, P. (1996) *The Lives to Come: the genetic revolution and human possibilities*. New York: Simon and Schuster.

Knill, P. J. (2004) *Principles and Practice of Expressive Arts Therapy: toward a therapeutic aesthetics*. London: Jessica Kingsley.

Kronenberg, F. and Pollard, N. (2005) 'Overcoming occupational apartheid; a preliminary exploration of the political nature of occupational therapy', in F. Kronenberg, S. Algado and N. Pollard (eds) *Occupational Therapy Without Borders*. Oxford: Elsevier.

Kymlicka, A. (2001) *Politics in the Vernacular: Nationalism, Multiculturalism and Citizenship*. Oxford: Oxford University Press.

Laing, R. D. (1967) *The Politics of Experience and the Bird of Paradise*. Harmondsworth: Penguin.

Lapper, A. (2005) *My Life in My Hands*. London: Simon and Schuster.

Langan, M. (1998) 'Radical social work' in R. Adams, L. Dominelli and M. Payne (eds) *Social Work: themes, issues and debates*. London: Macmillan.

Langan. M. and Lee, P. (1989) *Radical Social Work Today*. London: Routledge.

Lawnmowers (2006) Publicity material. Newcastle upon Tyne.

Lenaghan, J. (1998) *Brave New NHS? The impact of human genetics on the health service.* London: Institute for Public Policy Research.

Leonard, P. (1997) *Postmodern Welfare: reconstructing an emancipatory project.* London: Sage.

Linton, S. (1998) *Claiming Disability: knowledge and identity.* New York. New York Disability Press.

'Living with Aids: Britain's battle' (2006) BBC Radio 4. 4 November.

Longmore, P.K. and Umansky, L. (eds) (2001) *The New Disability History.* New York: New York University Press.

Lonsdale, S. (1990) *Women and Disability.* London: Macmillan.

Looking Beyond Labels: widening the opportunity for employment for people with disabilities in the new NHS (2001) London: Department of Health.

Macfarlane, A. (1994) 'Watershed', in L. Keith (ed.) *Mustn't Crumble: writing by disabled women.* London: The Women's Press.

MacFie, J., Cicchetti, D. and Toth, S. (2001) 'Dissociation in maltreated versus non-maltreated preschool-aged children', *Child Abuse and Neglect,* 25: 1253–1267.

Maheady D.C. (2003) *Nursing Students with Disabilities Change the Course.* River Edge, NJ: Exceptional Parent Press.

Maheady D.C. (2006) *Leave No Nurse Behind: nurses working with disabilities.* New York: Universe INC.

Malin, N. (1983) *Group Homes for the Mentally Handicapped.* London: HMSO.

Manco-Johnson, M., Morrissey-Harding, G., Edelman-Lewis, B. & Oster, G. (2004) 'Development and validation of a measure of disease specific quality of life in young children with haemophilia', *Haemophilia,* 10: 34–41.

Markova, I. & Forbes, C. (1984) 'Coping with haemophilia', *International Review of Applied Psychology,* 33: 457–477.

Marks, D. (1999) *Disability: controversial debates and psychosocial perspectives.* London: Routledge.

Martin, J.P. (1984) *Hospitals in Trouble.* Oxford: Basil Blackwell.

Mason, M. (2000) *Incurably Human.* London: Working Press.

Mathews, D.R. (1997) 'The OK health check: a health assessment checklist for people with learning disabilities', *British Journal of Learning Disabilities,* 25: 139–143.

McGee, J. and Menolascino, F. (1991) *Beyond Gentle Teaching: a non-aversive approach to helping those in need.* London: Plenum Press.

McGee, J., Menolascino, F., Hobbs, D. and Menousek, P (1987) *Gentle Teaching: a non-aversive approach to helping people with mental retardation.* New York: Human Sciences Press.

McIver, R. (2005) 'Crossing the Jungle in a Wheelchair'. http://news.bbc.co.uk/1/hi/health/4319920.stm (17 November)

McKnight, J. (1978) 'Professionalised services and disabling help', in I. Illich, I. Zola, J. McKnight, J. Caplan and H. Saiken (eds) *Disabling Professions.* London: Marion Boyars.

McKnight, J. (1995) *The Careless Society: community and its counterfeits.* New York: Basic.

Mencap (1997) *Prescription for Change (Summary).* London: Mencap Research.

Menzel, P., Dolan, P., Richardson, J. & Olsen, J. A. (2002) 'The role of adaptation to disability and disease in health state valuation: a preliminary normative analysis', *Social Science and Medicine,* 55, 2149–2158.

Mercer, G. (2004) 'User-Led Organisations: facilitation independent living', in J. Swain, S. French, C. Barnes and C. Thomas (eds) (2004) *Disabling Barriers – Enabling Environments,* 2nd edn. London: Sage.

Michalko, R. (2002) *The Difference that Disability Makes*. Philadelphia: Temple University Press.

Mickery, L. (2004) *Every Time You Look at Me*. www.bbc.co.uk/drama (10 May).

Middleton, L. (1992) *Children First: working with children and disability*. Birmingham: Venture Press.

Miller, N.B. and Sammons, C.C. (1999) *Everybody's Different: understanding and changing our reactions to disabilities*. London: Paul Brookes.

Mills, C.W. (1956) *The Power Elite*. Oxford: Oxford University Press.

Milton, J. (2003) The Major Works (Oxford World's Classics). Oxford: Oxford University Press.

Miners, A., Sabin, C., Tolley, K., Jenkinson, C., Kind, P. & Lee, C. (1999) 'Assessing health-related quality-of-life in individuals with haemophilia', *Haemophilia*, 5: 378–385.

Minty, S. (2004) 'Interview with Alison Walsh', (11 May) *Disability World: A Bimonthly Webzine of International Disability News and Views*, 5 (October–December 2000) www.disabilityworld.org.

Mitchell, D. (2006) Introduction. In Mitchell, D., Traustadottir, R., Townson, L., Ingham, N. and Ledger, S. (eds) *Exploring Experiences of Advocacy by People with Learning Disabilities: testimonies of resistance*. London: Jessica Kingsley.

Mitchell, M. (1994) 'Epilepsy: self-portraits of sigmatisation', *DAM*, 4 (Autumn).

Mocellin, G. (1996) 'Occupational therapy: a critical overview, part 2', *British Journal of Occupational Therapy*, 59(1): 11–16.

Modern American Poetry website: http://www.english.uiuc.edu/maps/poets/a_f/brown/oldlem.htm (visited 01 October 2006).

Mohlo, P., Rolland, N., Lebrun, T., Dirat, G., Courpied, J., Croughs, T., Duprat, I., Sutlan, Y. & The French Study Group (2000) 'Epidemiological survey of the orthopaedic status of severe haemophilia A and B patients in France', *Haemophilia*, 6: 23–32.

Monks, J. (1999) "It works both ways": belonging and social participation among women with disabilities', in N. Yuval-Davis and P. Werbner (eds) *Women, Citizenship and Difference*. London: Zed Books.

Morgan, D. (1997) *Focus Groups as Qualitative Research*. London: Sage.

Morris, J. (1989) *Able Lives: women's experience of paralysis*. London: The Women's Press.

Morris, J. (1991) *Pride against Prejudice: a personal politics of disability*. London: The Women's Press.

Morris, S. (2006) 'Twisted lies: my journey in an imperfect body', in E. Parens (ed.) *Surgically Shaping Children: technology, ethics and the pursuit of normality*. Baltimore: Johns Hopkins University Press.

Mullen, P., Martin, J.L., Anderson, J.C., Romans, S.E. and Herbison, G.P. (1994) 'The effect of child sexual abuse on social, interpersonal and sexual function in adult life', *British Journal of Psychiatry*, 165: 35–47.

Muller, H.J. (1936) *Out of the Night: a biologist's view of the future*. London: Victor Gollancz.

Murray, P. and Penman, J. (1996) *Let Our Children Be: a collection of stories*. Sheffield: Parents with Attitude.

Murray, P. and Penman, J. (2000) *Telling our Stories: reflections on family life in a disabling world*. Sheffield: Parents with Attitude.

Nairne, S. (2004) www.fourthplinth.co.uk/press_release 16 June

Neath J. and Schriner K. (1998) 'power to people with disabilities: empowerment issues in employment planning', *Disability and society*, 13(3): 217–228.

Newman, E., Kaloupek, D., Keane, T. and Folstein, S. (1997) 'Ethical issues in trauma research: the evolution of an empirical model for decision making', in G. Kaufman Kantor and J. Jasinski (eds) *Out of the Darkness: contemporary perspectives on family violence*. Thousand Oaks, CA: Sage.

NHS Direct (2006) *NHS Careers*. London: Department of Health (www.nhscareers.nhs.uk).

Noakes, V. (ed.) (2001) *Edward Lear: the complete verse and other nonsense*. Harmondsworth: Penguin.

Norden, M.F. (1994) *The Cinema of Isolation – A History of Physical Disability in the Movies*. New Brunswick, NJ: Rutgers University Press.

Norman, J. (2000) 'Constructive narrative in arresting the impact of post-traumatic stress disorder', *Clinical Social Work Journal*, 28(3): 303–319.

Nunkoosing, K. (2000) 'Constructing learning disability: consequences for men and women with learning disabilities', *Journal of Learning Disabilities*, 14(1): 46–62.

Nursing and Midwifery Council (NMC) (2006) *Fitness to Practice*, London: Nursing & Midwifery Council.

Ochs, E. and Capps, L. (1996) 'Narrating the self', *Annual Review of Anthropology*, 25: 19–43.

Oliver, M. (1986) 'Social policy and disability: some theoretical issues', *Disability, Handicap and Society*, 1(1): 5–17.

Oliver, M. (1990) *The Politics of Disablement*. Basingstoke: Macmillan.

Oliver, M. (1993a) 'Disability: a creation of industrialised societies?' in J. Swain, V. Finkelstein, S. French and M. Oliver (eds) *Disabling Barriers: Enabling Environments*. Buckingham: Open University Press.

Oliver, M. (1993b) 'Disability and dependency: a creation of industrial societies', in J. Swain, V. Finkelstein, S. French and M. Oliver (eds) *Disabling Barriers – Enabling Environments*. London: Sage.

Oliver, M. (1996) *Understanding Disability: from theory to practice*. Basingstoke: Macmillan.

Oliver, M. (2004) 'If I had a hammer: the social model in action', in J. Swain, S. French, C. Barnes and C. Thomas (eds) *Disabling Barriers – Enabling Environments*. London: Sage.

Oliver, M. and Barnes, C. (1996) *Disabled People and Social Policy: from exclusion to inclusion*. London: Longman.

Oliver, M. and Sapey, B. (1999) *Social Work with Disabled People*, 2nd edn. Basingstoke: Macmillan.

Olsen, R. and Clarke, H. (2003) *Parenting and Disability: disabled people's experiences of raising children*. Bristol: The Policy Press.

Onken, S. and Slaten, E. (2000) 'Disability identity formation and affirmation: the experiences of a person with severe mental illness', *Sociological Practice: A Journal of Clinical and Applied Sociology*, 2(2): 99–111.

Ostman, R. (1996) 'Photography and persuasion; farm security administration photographs of circus and carnival sideshows, 1935–1942', in R. Garland Thomson (ed.) *Freakery: cultural spectacles of the extraordinary body*. New York: New York University Press.

Oswin, M. (1973) *The Empty Hours: a study of the weekend life of handicapped children in institutions*. London: Penguin.

O'Toole, R., Webster, S.W., O'Toole, A.W. and Lucal, B. (1999) 'Teachers' recognition and reporting of child abuse: a factorial survey', *Child Abuse and Neglect*, 23(11): 1083–1101.

Panagos, J. (1996) 'Speech therapy discourse: the input to learning', in M. Smith and J. Damico (eds) *Childhood Language Disorders*. New York: Thieme.

Parens, E. and Asch, A. (2000a) 'The disability rights critique of prenatal genetic testing: reflections and recommendations', in E. Parens and A. Asch (eds) *Prenatal Testing and Disability Rights*. Washington, DC: Georgetown University Press.

Parens, E. and Asch, A. (eds) (2000b) *Prenatal Testing and Disability Rights*. Washington, DC: Georgetown University Press.

Park, D.C. and Radford, J.P. (1999) 'From the case files: reconstructing a history of involuntary sterilisation', *Disability and Society*, 13(3): 317–342.

Park, J., Scott, K. & Benseman, J. (1999) 'Dealing with a bleeding nuisance: a study of haemophilia care in New Zealand', *New Zealand Medical Journal*, 112: 155–158.

Parr, S., Duchan, J. and Pound, C. (2003) *Aphasia Inside Out*. Maidenhead: Open University Press.

Parr, S., Pound, C. and Hewitt, A. (2006) Communication access to health and social services, *Topics in Language Disorders*, 26: 189–198.

Patten, B. (1981) *Clare's Countryside: natural history poetry and prose by John Clare*. London: Heinemann Quixote Press.

Paul, D. (1992) 'Eugenic anxieties, social realities and political choices', *Social Research*, 59(3): 663–683.

Pearlin, L. & Schooler, C. (1978) 'The structure of coping', *Journal of Health and Social Behavior*, 19: 2–21.

Peters, S. (2000) 'Is there a disability culture? Some theoretical issues', *Disability and Society*, 15(4): 583–601.

Phillips, A. and Daniluk, J. (2004) 'Beyond "survivor": how childhood sexual abuse informs the identity of adult women at the end of the therapeutic process', *Journal of Counselling and Development*, 82(2): 177–184.

Plummer, K. (1995) *Telling Sexual Stories: power, change and social worlds*. London: Routledge.

Poe, E.A. (1917) *Eleonora, The Fall of the House of Usher & The Purloined Letter*. New York: P.F. Collier & Son.

Pointon, A. and Davies, C. (1997) *Framed: interrogating disability in the media*. London: British Film Institute.

Pollard, N., Alsop, A. and Kroneberg, F. (2005) 'Reconceptualising occupational therapy', *British Journal of Occupational Therapy*, 68(11): 524–526.

Pope, A. (1961) 'Prologue to the Satires', in A. Pope, *Epistles and Satires*. Houndsmill: Macmillan.

Potts, M. and Fido, R. (1991) *'A Fit Person To Be Removed': personal accounts of life in a mental deficiency institution*. Plymouth: Northcote House.

Pound, C. (2004) 'Dare to be different: the person and the practice', in S. Byng and J. Duchan (eds) *Challenging Aphasia Therapies*. London: Psychology Press.

Pound, C. and Hewitt, A. (2004) 'Communication barriers: building access and identity', in J. Swain, S. French, C. Barnes and C. Thomas (eds) (2004) *Disabling Barriers – Enabling Environments*, 2nd edn. London: Sage.

Priestley, M. (1995) 'Dropping 'E's: the missing link in quality assurance for disabled people', *Critical Social Policy*, 44: 7–21.

Priestley, M. (1999) *Disability Politics and Community Care*. London: Jessica Kingsley.

Pring, J. (2003) *Silent Victims*. London: Gibson Square Books.

Provus McElroy, L. (1992) 'Early indicators of pathological dissociation in sexually abused children', *Child Abuse and Neglect*, 16: 833–846.

Pultz, J. (1995) *Photography and the Body.* London: Weidenfeld and Nicolson.

Quinn, M. (2002) *Tate Liverpool Catalogue.*

Ramcharan, P. (ed.) (1997) *Empowerment in Everyday Life: learning difficulties.* London: Jessica Kingsley.

Richardson, A. and Richardson, J. (1989) *Enabling People with Learning Difficulties to Make and Maintain Friends.* London: Policy Studies Institute.

Ridley, M. (2006) *Francis Crick: discoverer of the genetic code.* London: HarperCollins.

Reilly, M. (1958) 'An occupational therapy curriculum for 1965', *American Journal of Occupational Therapy*, 12(6): 293–299.

Reynolds, F. (2004) 'The subjective experience of illness', in S. French & J. Sim (eds) *Physiotherapy-a psychosocial approach.* 3rd edn. London: Butterworth Heinemann.

Richards, T. & Richards, L. (1998) Using computers in qualitative research. In N. Denzin, & Y. Lincoln (eds) *Collecting and Interpreting Qualitative Methods.* London: Sage.

Rizza, C. (1997) Clinical features and diagnosis of haemophilia, Christmas disease and von Willebrand's disease. In C. Rizza & G. Lowe (eds) *Haemophilia and Other Inherited Bleeding Disorders.* London: W. B. Saunders and Company Ltd.

Robert, S.A. and House, J.S. (2000) 'Socioeconomic inequalities in health: integrating individual-community and societal-level theory and research', in G.L. Albrecht, R. Fitzpatrick and S.C. Scrimshaw (eds) *The Handbook of Social Studies in Health and Medicine.* London: Sage.

Rogers, L. (1999) 'Having disabled babies will be 'sin' says scientist', *Sunday Times*, 4 July.

Rolfe, G., Freshwater, D. and Jasper, M. (2001) *Critical reflection for nursing and the helping professions: a user's guide.* Basingstoke: Palgrave.

Rorty, R. (1999) *Philosophy and Social Hope.* London: Penguin.

Rose, N. (1985) *The Psychological Complex.* London: Routledge.

Rosendaal, F., Smit, C., Varekamp, I., Brocker-Vriends, A., Van Dijck, H., Suurmeijer, T., Vandenbroucke, J. & Briet, E. (1990) 'Modern haemophilia treatment: medical improvements and quality of life', *Journal of Internal Medicine*, 228: 633–640.

Rosenhan, D. L. (1973) 'On being sane in insane places', *Science*, 179: 250–258.

Royal College of Nursing (2003) *Workability 2: Information for RCN representatives, employers and injured, ill or disabled nurses: Getting on with the job!* London: Royal College of Nursing.

Royal, S., Schramm, W., Berntorp E., Giangrande, P., Gringeri, A., Ludlum C., Kroner B. & Szacs T. (2002) 'Quality of life differences between prophylactic and on demand factor replacement therapy in European haemophilia patients', *Haemophilia*, 8: 33–43.

Russell, M. (1998) *Beyond Ramps: disability at the end of the social contract.* Monroe: Common Courage Press.

Ryan, J. and Thomas, F. (1987) *The Politics of Mental Handicap.* London: Free Association.

Ryan, W. (1971) *Blaming the Victim.* London: Orbach and Chambers.

Salaman, G. (1979) *Work Organisations, Resistance and Control.* London: Routledge and Kegan Paul.

Salk, L., Hilgartner, M. & Granich, B. (1972) 'The psycho-social impact of hemophilia on the patient and his family', *Social Science and Medicine*, 6: 491–505.

Saraga, E. and MacLeod, M. (1997) 'False memory syndrome: theory or defence against reality?' *Feminism and Psychology*, 7(1): 46–51.

Saxton, M. (2000) 'Why members of the disability community oppose prenatal diagnosis and selective abortion', in E. Parens and A. Asch (eds) *Prenatal Testing and Disability Rights.* Washington, DC: Georgetown University Press.

Seedhouse, D. (2001) *Health: the foundations for achievement,* 2nd edn. Chichester: John Wiley and Sons.

Shakespeare, T. (1994) 'Cultural representation of disabled people: dustbins for disavowal?' *Disability and Society,* 9(3): 283–299.

Shakespeare, T. (1999) 'Losing the plot? Medical and activist discourses of contemporary genetics and disability', *Sociology of Health and Illness,* 21(5): 669–688.

Shakespeare, T. (2005) 'The social context of reproductive choices', in D. Wasserman, J. Bickenbach and R. Wachbroit (eds) *Quality of Life and Human Difference: genetic testing, healthcare and disability.* Cambridge: Cambridge University Press.

Shakespeare, T. (2006) *Disability Rights and Wrongs.* London: Routledge.

Shakespeare, T., Gillespie-Sells, K. and Davies, D. (1996) *The Sexual Politics of Disability.* London: Cassell.

Shakespeare, W. (2000) *The Complete Works.* London: J. M. Dent.

Shamash, M. (2005) 'Review of Frida Kahlo exhibition', *Disability Now,* July.

Sidell, M. (1993) Interpreting. In P. Shakespeare, D. Atkinson & S. French (eds) *Reflecting on Research Practice.* Buckingham: Open University Press.

Simmons-Mackie, N. and Damico, J. (1999) 'Social role negotiation in aphasia therapy: competence, incompetence and conflict', in D. Kovarsky, J. Duchan and M. Maxwell (eds) *Constructing (In)Competence.* New Jersey: Lawrence Erlbaum.

Simon, D. (1998) *Guiding Recovery from Child Sexual Abuse.* London: Jessica Kingsley.

Sinclair, K. (2005) 'Foreword', in F. Kronenberg, S.S. Algado and N. Pollard (eds) *Occupational Therapy Without Borders.* Oxford: Elsevier.

Sinson, J. (1994) 'Normalisation and community integration of adults with mental handicap relocated to group homes', *Journal of Developmental and Physical Disabilities,* 6(3): 225–270.

Smith, R. (2006) 'Our baby twins were designed to be healthy', *London Lite,* November: 19.

Snyder, S.L. and Mitchell, D.T. (2006a) *Cultural Locations of Disability.* Chicago: University of Chicago Press.

Snyder, S.L. and Mitchell, D.T. (2006b) 'Eugenics', in G.A. Albrecht (ed.) *Encyclopedia of Disability.* London: Sage.

Solomon, J. (1992) 'Child sexual abuse by family members: a radical feminist perspective', *Sex Roles,* 27(9/10): 473–485.

Solovieva, S. (2001) 'Clinical severity of disease, functional disability and health-related quality of life: three year follow-up study of 150 Finnish patients with coagulation disorders', *Haemophilia,* 7: 53–63.

Spence, D. (1982) *Narrative Truth and Historical Truth: meaning and interpretation in psycho-analysis.* London: W.W. Norton.

Stacey, M. (1992) *Regulating British Medicine: The General Medical Council.* Chichester: John Wiley and Sons.

Stiker, H. (1997) *A History of Disability.* Ann Arbor: University of Michigan Press.

Stone, E. (1999a) 'Disability and development in the majority world', in E. Stone (ed.) *Disability and Development: learning from action and research on disability in the majority world.* Leeds: The Disability Press.

Stone, E. (1999b) 'Modern slogan, ancient script: impairment and disability in the Chinese language', in M. Corker and S. French (eds) *Disability Discourse.* Buckingham: Open University Press.

Straughair, S. and Fawcitt, S. (1992) *The Road Towards Independence: the experiences of young people with arthritis in the 1990s.* London: Arthritis Care.

Sullivan, J. and Beech, A. (2002) 'Professional perpetrators: sex offenders who use their employment to target and sexually abuse the children with whom they work', *Child Abuse Review*, 1(3): 153–167.

Sullivan, P. and Knutson, J. (2000) 'Maltreatment and disabilities: a population based epidemiological study', *Child Abuse and Neglect*, 24(10): 1257–1273.

Sumison, T. (1999) *Implementation Issues: Client-Centred Practice In Occupational Therapy*. Edinburgh: Churchill Livingston.

Summit, R. (1983) 'The child sexual abuse accommodation syndrome', *Child Abuse and Neglect*, 7: 177–193.

Sutherland, A. (1995) *Chronology of Disability Arts*. London: Edward Lear Foundation. Online at http://www.disabilityarts.com/.

Sutherland, A.T. (1981) *Disabled We Stand*. London: Souvenir Press.

Swain, J., Gillman, M. and French, S. (1998) *Confronting Disabling Barriers: towards making organisations accessible*. Birmingham: Venture Press.

Swain, J. and Cameron, C. (1999) 'Unless otherwise stated: discourses of labelling and identity in coming out', in M. Corker and S. French (eds) *Disability Discourse*. Buckingham: Open University Press.

Swain, J. and French, S. (2000) 'Towards an affirmation model of disability', *Disability and Society*, 15(4): 569–582.

Swain, J. and French, S. (2004) 'Researching together: a participatory approach', in S. French and J. Sim (eds) *Physiotherapy: a psychosocial approach*. Oxford: Butterworth-Heinemann.

Swain J., French, S., Barnes, C. and Thomas, C. (eds) (2004) *Disabling Barriers – Enabling Environments*, 2nd edn. London: Sage.

Swain, J., Finkelstein, V., French, S and Oliver, M. (eds) (1993) *Disabling Barriers – Enabling Environments*. London: Sage.

Swain, J., Heyman, B. and Gillman, M. (1998) 'Public research, private concerns: ethical issues in the use of open-ended interviews with people who have learning difficulties', *Disability and Society*, 13(1): 21–36.

Swain, J., French, S. and Cameron, C. (2003) *Controversial Issues in a Disabling Society*. Buckingham: Open University Press.

Swinburn, K. (2005) 'Journeys with aphasia: personal reflections', in C. Anderson and A. van der Gaag (eds) *Speech and Language Therapy Issues in Professional Practice*. London: Whurr.

Tackling Attitudes of Healthcare Professionals Towards Disabled people (2005) *University of Bristol News*, University of Bristol Press, 3 October.

Taylor, S. (1983) 'Adjustment to threatening events: a theory of cognitive adaptation', *American Psychologist*, 38, 1161–1173.

Taylor, D. (1989) 'Citizenship and social power', *Critical Social Policy*, 26: 19–31.

'Thalidomide: 40 Years On' (2002) BBC Radio 4. 7 June.

Thomas, C. (1998) 'Parents and families: disabled women's stories about their childhood experiences', in C. Robinson and K. Stalker (eds) *Growing Up with Disability*. London: Jessica Kingsley.

Thomas, C. (1999) *Female Forms: experiencing and understanding disability*. Buckingham: Open University Press.

Thompson, N. (1998) *Promoting Equality*. Basingstoke: Macmillan Press.

Thompson, J. and Pickering, S (2001) *Meeting the Health Needs of People Who Have a Learning Disability*. London: Bailliere Tindall.

Thompson, N. (2001) *Anti-discriminatory Practice*, 3rd edn. Houndmills: Palgrave.

Thomson, M. (1998) *The Problem of Mental Deficiency Eugenics, Democracy and Social Policy in Britain*. Oxford: Clarendon Press.

Townsend, E. (1993) 'Muriel Driver lecture: occupational therapy's social vision', *Canadian Journal of Occupational Therapy*. 60(4): 174–184.

Townsend, E. and Brintell, S.S. (1997) 'Context of occupational therapy', in E. Townsend, S. Stanton, M. Law, P. Polatajako, S. Baptiste, T. Thompson- Franson, K. Kramer, F. Swedlove, L. Britnell and L. Campanelle (eds) *Enabling Occupation: an occupational perspective*. Ottawa: CAOT Publications.

Townsend, E. and Wilcock, A.A. (2004) 'Occupational justice and client-centred practice: a dialogue in progress', *Canadian Journal of Occupational Therapy*, 71(2): 75–87.

Trippoli, S., Viaiani, M., Linari, S., Longo, G., Morfini, M. & Messori, A. (2001) 'Multivariate analysis of factors influencing quality of life and utility in patients with haemophilia', *Hemostasis and Thrombosis*, 86: 722–728.

Tyneside Disability Arts (1998) *Sub Rosa*. Wallsend: TDA.

Tyneside Disability Arts (1999) *Transgressions*. Wallsend: TDA.

University of Bristol News (2005) *Partners in Practice: Disability Equality*. www.bris.ac.uk/news/

UPIAS (1972) 'Contribution to the discussion on the nature of our organization': extract from *UPIAS Circular, 3* (c. December).

Van der Gaag, A. and Anderson, C. (2005) 'The geography of professional practice: swamps and icebergs', in C. Anderson and A. van der Gaag (eds) *Speech and Language Therapy Issues in Professional Practice*. London: Whurr.

Van der Gaag, A. and Mowles. C. (2005) 'Values in professional practice', in C. Anderson and A. van der Gaag (eds) *Speech and Language Therapy Issues in Professional Practice*. London: Whurr.

van der Kolk, B. and van der Hart, O. (1991) 'The intrusive past: the flexibility of memory and the engraving of trauma', *American Image*, 48: 425–454.

Vasey, S. (1992) 'Disability culture: it's a way of life', in R. Rieser and M. Mason (eds) *Disability Equality in the Classroom: a human rights issue*. London: Disability Equality in Education.

Vernon, A. (1999) 'The dialectics of multiple identities and the disabled people's movement', *Disability and Society*, 14(3): 385–398.

Vernon, A. and Swain, J. (2002) 'Theorizing divisions and hierarchies: towards a commonality or diversity?' in C. Barnes, M. Oliver and L. Barton (eds) *Disability Studies Today*. Cambridge: Polity Press.

Vondra, J. and Belsky, F. (1993) 'Developmental origins of parenting: personality and relationship factors', in T. Luster and L. Okagaki (eds) *Parenting: an ecological perspective*. Hillsdale, NJ: Lawrence Erlbaum Associates.

Waddington Street Writers (1997) *Light from a Black Hole*. London: Waddington Street Writers Group.

Wald, N. et al. (1992) 'Antenatal maternal screening for Down's syndrome: results of a demonstration project', *British Medical Journal*, 305: 391–394.

Walton, R. (2005) 'Social work as social institution', *British Journal of Social Work*, 35: 587–607.

Wang, T., Zhang, L., Li, H., Zhao, H. & Yang, R. (2004) 'Assessing health-related quality-of-life in individuals with haemophilia in China', *Haemophilia*, 10: 370–375.

Ward, L. (ed.) (2001) *Considered Choices: the new genetics, prenatal testing and people with learning disabilities*. Kidderminster: British Institute of Learning Disabilities.

Wardhaugh, J. and Wilding, P. (1993) 'Towards an explanation of the corruption of care', *Critical Social Policy*, 13: 4–31.

Wates, M. (1997) *Supporting Disabled Adults in their Parenting Role*. Oxford: NCT and Radcliffe Medical Press.

Watson, J.D. (2000) *A Passion for DNA: genes, genomes and society*. Oxford: Oxford University Press.

Watson, N. (2002) 'Well, I know it is going to sound strange to you, but I don't see myself as a disabled person: identity and disability', *Disability and Society*, 17(5): 509–527.

Wendell, S. (1996) *The Rejected Body: feminist philosophical reflections on disability*. New York: Routledge.

Wendell, S. (1997) 'Towards a feminist theory of disability', in J.L. Davis (ed.) *The Disability Studies Reader*. London: Routledge.

Wertz, D. (1999) 'Eugenics is alive and well: a survey of genetics professionals around the world', *Science in Context*, 11(3): 493–510.

Westcott, H. and Jones, D. (1999) 'Annotation: the abuse of disabled children', *Journal of Child Psychology and Psychiatry*, 40(4): 497–506.

Wetherell, M. and Maybin, J. (1997) 'The distributed self: a social constructionist perspective', in R. Stevens (ed.) *Understanding the Self*. London: Sage/Open University.

Wilcock, A.A. (2000). Development of a personal, professional and educational occupational philosophy: An Australian perspective. *Occupational Therapy International*, 7, 1-6. Retrieved May 14, 2002, from the Proquest database.

Wilder, E. (2006) *Wheeling and Dealing: living with spinal cord injury*. Nashville: Vanderbilt University Press.

Williams, J. (1993) 'What is a profession? Experience versus expertise', in J. Walmsley, J. Reynolds, P. Shakespeare and R. Woolfe (eds) *Health, Welfare and Practice: reflecting on roles and relationships*. London: Sage.

Williams, S. (2000) 'Chronic illness as biographical disruption or biographical disruption as chronic illness? Reflections on a core concept', *Sociology of Health and Illness*, 22: 4–67.

Wiseman, R. (2004) *The Luck Factor*. London: Arrow.

Wolfensberger, W. (1972) *The Principle of Normalisation in Human Services*. Toronto: National Institute on Mental Retardation.

Woodward, K. (2000) 'Questions of identity', in K. Woodward (ed.) *Questioning Identity: Gender, Class Nation*. London: Routledge.

Working Well Initiative (2002) London: Royal College of Nursing.

Wright D. (2000) 'Educational support for nursing and midwifery students with dyslexia', *Nursing Standard*, 28: (41): 35–41.

Wright, C. and Rowe, N. (2005) 'Protecting professional identities: service user involvement and occupational therapy', *British Journal of Occupational Therapy*, 68(1): 45–47.

Young, I. M. (1990) *Justice and the Politics of Difference*. Princeton, NJ: Princeton University Press.

Young, L. (1992) 'Sexual abuse and the problem of embodiment', *Child Abuse and Neglect*, 16: 89–100.

Young, N., Bradley, C., Blanchette, V., Wakefield, C., Barnard, D., Wu, J. & McCusker, P. (2004) 'Development of a health-related quality of life measure for boys with haemophilia: the Canadian Haemophilia Outcomes – Kids Life Assessment Tool (CHO-KLAT)', *Haemophilia*, 10: 34–43.

Younger, J. (1991) 'A theory of mastery', *Advances in Nursing Science*, 14: 76–89.

Index